EYE AND VISION RESEARCH DEVELOPMENTS

GLAUCOMA:
ETIOLOGY, PATHOGENESIS
AND TREATMENTS

EYE AND VISION
RESEARCH DEVELOPMENTS

Additional books in this series can be found on Nova's website
under the Series tab.

Additional E-books in this series can be found on Nova's website
under the E-book tab.

EYE AND VISION RESEARCH DEVELOPMENTS

GLAUCOMA: ETIOLOGY, PATHOGENESIS AND TREATMENTS

Z.G. FEI

AND

SEIJI ZENG

EDITORS

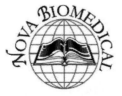

Nova Biomedical Books
New York

For permission to use material from this book please contact us:
Telephone 631-231-7269; Fax 631-231-8175
Web Site: http://www.novapublishers.com

NOTICE TO THE READER

The Publisher has taken reasonable care in the preparation of this book, but makes no expressed or implied warranty of any kind and assumes no responsibility for any errors or omissions. No liability is assumed for incidental or consequential damages in connection with or arising out of information contained in this book. The Publisher shall not be liable for any special, consequential, or exemplary damages resulting, in whole or in part, from the readers' use of, or reliance upon, this material. Any parts of this book based on government reports are so indicated and copyright is claimed for those parts to the extent applicable to compilations of such works.

Independent verification should be sought for any data, advice or recommendations contained in this book. In addition, no responsibility is assumed by the publisher for any injury and/or damage to persons or property arising from any methods, products, instructions, ideas or otherwise contained in this publication.

This publication is designed to provide accurate and authoritative information with regard to the subject matter covered herein. It is sold with the clear understanding that the Publisher is not engaged in rendering legal or any other professional services. If legal or any other expert assistance is required, the services of a competent person should be sought. FROM A DECLARATION OF PARTICIPANTS JOINTLY ADOPTED BY A COMMITTEE OF THE AMERICAN BAR ASSOCIATION AND A COMMITTEE OF PUBLISHERS.

Additional color graphics may be available in the e-book version of this book.

LIBRARY OF CONGRESS CATALOGING-IN-PUBLICATION DATA

ISBN: 978-1-61470-975-6

Library of Congress Control Number: 2011029487

Published by Nova Science Publishers, Inc. † New York

Contents

Preface

Glaucoma is an eye disorder in which the optic nerve suffers damage, permanently damaging vision in the affected eye(s) and progressing to complete blindness if untreated. It is often, but not always, associated with increased pressure of the fluid in the eye. In this book, the authors present topical research in the study of the etiology, pathogenesis and treatments of glaucoma. Topics discussed in this compilation include medical treatment in chronic open-angle glaucoma; melatonin as a therapeutic resource for the management of glaucoma; ocular tissue changes and glaucoma treatment; secondary uveitic glaucoma; selective laser trabeculoplasty and parasurgical treatment of glaucoma.

Chapter I - It is a well-known fact that the term glaucoma covers a wide range of progressive optic neuropathies characterized by a specific pattern of optic nerve head and visual field damage. Additionally, it is also known, that the key goal in glaucoma therapy should be preserving vision and the patient`s quality of life.Persistent elevated intraocular pressure is probably the most important risk factor for the development and progression of glaucoma, but it is still a risk factor and not a disease per se. Over the past few years, with the introduction of newer drugs, there has been a gradual shift in the choice of medical therapy. Currently available options for medical treatment of chronic open-angle glaucoma include topical Beta adrenergic blocking agents, adrenergic drugs, miotics, carbonic anhydrase inhibitors, and prostaglandin analogues/prostamides. Ophthalmology community has welcomed the increase in the variety of therapeutic options for the authors' patients. However, at the same time, it has become more confused the election between the different monotherapies and the fixed or unfixed combination options. Medical therapy as a rule starts with one drug. Nevertheless, the choice of management strategy must take into account efficacy, safety, tolerability, quality of life, adherence, and cost. Additionally, it is important when selecting the medical treatment of glaucoma to understand not only the aims of therapy but also the mode of action, side effects, and contraindications of each individual medication. Finally, it is essential to realized that preservatives contained within topical eye drop preparations may cause inflammatory conjunctival side effects and toxicity on the ocular surface. The use of preservative-free medications may be considered to avoid such problems.

Chapter II - Glaucoma is a complex disease with a number of risk factors and mechanisms which lead to retinal ganglion cell (RGC) death. Ocular hypertension is probably the most important risk factor for primary angle open glaucoma, the more frequent form of glaucoma. However, other factors such as excitotoxicity, reduced antioxidant defense system activity, and an increase in the nitridergic pathway activity have been suggested as possible additional causes for glaucomatous damage. The current management of glaucoma is mainly directed at the control of intraocular pressure (IOP); however, a therapy that prevents the death of RGCs and optic nerve head fiber loss should be the main goal of treatment. In recent years, melatonin has been identified as a neuroprotector in experimental animal models of various neurological and neurodegenerative disorders. In this chapter, the authors will consider evidence supporting that melatonin, a very safe compound for human use, should be regarded as a new therapeutic resource for the management of glaucoma.

Chapter III - Primary open angle glaucoma (POAG) is the leading cause of irreversible and preventable visual field loss. Glaucoma is responsible for 14% of blindness worldwide and it is the second cause of blindness after cataract [1]. In the world, the primary glaucoma afflicts about 60-70 million people, of whom 10% are believed to be bilaterally blind [2,3,4]. POAG is characterized by a progressive optic neuropathy and it is usually asymptomatic until advanced. The most important risk factors include elevated intraocular pressure (IOP), positive family history, advanced age and African ancestry. The pathogenesis of glaucoma is not yet totally explained. POAG can occur with or without raised eye pressure, but nowadays an elevated intraocular pressure remains the main target to whom the authors can address the treatment: drugs, laser or surgery [5,6,7,8]. Glaucoma remains a major public health problem worldwide. Even in developed countries, half of glaucoma cases are undiagnosed until visual field changes arise. When the diagnosis of glaucoma has been made, patients need lifelong sight checking to prevent progression of visual field damage and to maintain a sighted lifetime. Glaucoma is commonly treated with daily eye-drop drugs to avoid the onset of further irreversible optic nerve damage and visual field defects [9].

Chapter IV - Secondary uveitic glaucoma is a common complication of intraocular inflammation and is present in up to 20% of patients with uveitis. The incidence of uveitis in the United States is estimated to be 200 cases per 100 000 people per year and mostly affects adults aged 20 to 50 years. This condition represents the fourth cause of legal blindness in patients between 20 and 60 years. Among the patients with uveitis visual loss occurs more frequently in patients with glaucoma than in patients without glaucoma. Several mechanisms are involved in the pathogenesis of uveitic glaucoma. It is clinically useful to classify it into 4 categories based on mechanism: inflammatory ocular hypertension syndrome; ocular hypertension due to acute uveitic angle closure; corticosteroid-induced ocular hypertension/glaucoma; and ocular hypertension/glaucoma due to chronic damage to aqueous outflow systems, most notably the trabecular meshwork. Uveitic glaucoma often gets worse despite intensive medical treatment, and it may require surgical intervention. Surgical management is challenging because of the increased risk of post-operative inflammation and failure to control intraocular pressure.

Chapter V - Selective laser trabeculoplasty (SLT) is a therapeutic modality that utilizes Neodymium: Yttrium aluminium garnet (Nd:YAG) laser to increase outflow facility in the trabecular meshwork(TM). It selectively targets pigmented cells in the trabecular meshwork causing little if any damage to trabecular cells. It presumably increases outflow facility by altering the composition of the extracellular matrix of the TM. SLT efficacy, safety, and repeatability have been extensively studied. SLT is equally effective to Argon Laser Trabeculoplasty (ALT) achieving on average a 20% reduction on intraocular pressure (IOP) despite causing significantly less histologic damage to TM. However, similarly to ALT SLT loses effectiveness over time and is occasionally accompanied by IOP spikes immediately after the procedure. SLT is effective irrespective of the amount of TM pigmentation and is particularly effective in secondary open angle glaucomas including pseudoexfoliation and pigmentary glaucoma. The only variable predictive of SLT success is IOP before the procedure. The major theoretical advantage of SLT over ALT is its potential for virtually limitless repeatability. However this advantage remains largely theoretical as there are few studies proving the efficacy of such repeatability. SLT is promising as single therapeutic intervention in third world countries because of the low rate of complications, the ease of application and the potential for repeat therapy. Although economic modeling has been used to advocate for widespread use in managed care environments, the economic advantages from a public health perspective in this setting are questionable.

Chapter VI - The treatment parasurgical of glaucoma classically occupies an intermediate place between the medical and surgical therapy and it is frequently used when the patient's particular conditions or specific forms of glaucoma, do not allow surgery. This type of therapy can be applied to the open-angle glaucoma (GPAA), acute glaucoma, and those glaucomas refractory to medical therapy and/or surgery.

Chapter VII - Purpose: To study hypotensive effect of synthetic cannabinoid WIN 55212-2 when topically administered at 0.5% and 1% concentration. The authors also studied the normal distribution of CB1 receptors in ocular tissues from rats. Matherials and controls: 24 female Sprague-Dawley rats, weighing between 250 and 300 g. Rats were divided in 6 groups according to the topical treatment for the left eye. Right eyes were considered as controls. Group 1: 0.5% WIN 55212-2, group 2: 1% WIN55212-2, group 3: 0.5% AM 251, group 4: 1% AM 251, group 5: 0.5% AM 251 and 0.5% WIN 55212-2, and group 6: 1% AM 251 and 1% WIN 55212-2. Intraocular pressure was measured in awake animals with applanation tonometry. Afterwards, control right eyes were employed for immunohistochemistry for CB1 receptors. Results: WIN 55212-2 0.5% induced an average decrease of 4±2.5 mm Hg (or 23.86±15.04%), with respect to the corresponding right eye. WIN 55212-2 1% solution-treated eyes showed an average decrease of 6.8±2 mm Hg (or 37.10±9.98%), and there was less fluctuation in the IOP tendencies of the treated eyes, with respect to the corresponding right eye. Hypotensive effect is abolished by previously topically application of CB1 antagonist AM251. CB1 antagonist AM 251 showed no effect on IOP. CB1 receptors were observed in the main therapeutic ocular targets for the treatment of glaucoma: trabecular meshwork, Schlemm's canal, nonpigmented epithelium of the ciliar body, and retina. Conclusions: WIN 55212-2 induce a dose-dependant intraocular hypotensive effect mainly through activation of CB1 receptors.

In: Glaucoma: Etiology, Pathogenesis and Treatments
Editors: Z. G. Fei and S. Zeng
ISBN: 978-1-61470-975-6
© 2012 Nova Science Publishers, Inc.

Chapter I

Medical Treatment in Chronic Open-Angle Glaucoma: An Update

Antonio Martinez Garcia[1] and Javier Benitez-del-Castillo[2]
[1]Science Ophthalmic Research
Address: Rosalia de Catsro, La Coruña),Spain
[2]Hospital General del S.A.S. de Jerez, Cadiz, Spain

ABSTRACT

It is a well-known fact that the term glaucoma covers a wide range of progressive optic neuropathies characterized by a specific pattern of optic nerve head and visual field damage. Additionally, it is also known, that the key goal in glaucoma therapy should be preserving vision and the patient's quality of life. Persistent elevated intraocular pressure is probably the most important risk factor for the development and progression of glaucoma, but it is still a risk factor and not a disease per se.

Over the past few years, with the introduction of newer drugs, there has been a gradual shift in the choice of medical therapy. Currently available options for medical treatment of chronic open-angle glaucoma include topical Beta adrenergic blocking agents, adrenergic drugs, miotics, carbonic anhydrase inhibitors, and prostaglandin analogues/prostamides.

Ophthalmology community has welcomed the increase in the variety of therapeutic options for our patients. However, at the same time, it has become more confused the election between the different monotherapies and the fixed or unfixed combination options.

Medical therapy as a rule starts with one drug. Nevertheless, the choice of management strategy must take into account efficacy, safety, tolerability, quality of life, adherence, and cost.

Additionally, it is important when selecting the medical treatment of glaucoma to understand not only the aims of therapy but also the mode of action, side effects, and contraindications of each individual medication.

Finally, it is essential to realized that preservatives contained within topical eye drop preparations may cause inflammatory conjunctival side effects and toxicity on the ocular surface. The use of preservative-free medications may be considered to avoid such problems.

1. INTRODUCTION

The term glaucoma covers a wide range of multifactorial, chronic, and progressive optic neuropathies characterized by a specific pattern of optic nerve head and visual field damage caused by a number of different diseases. Some of these diseases are becoming well characterized, whereas others, perhaps many, remain to be discovered or elucidated.

Treatment options for glaucoma include medications, laser therapy and incisional surgery. Laser techniques for the reduction of IOP include argon laser trabeculoplasty and selective laser trabeculoplasty.

It has long widely accepted that reduction of intraocular pressure is effective not only in preventing the onset of glaucoma [1, 2] but also in slowing the progression of glaucomatous damage [3-5]. In contrast, the available evidence does not suffice to determine which medical treatment or surgical procedure should be used as the first choice, or under what circumstances a patient who has been treated medically should undergo surgery.

For many years medical therapy has been the traditional initial modality of treatment to lower intraocular pressure in chronic open-angle glaucoma. It still is the standard initial therapy. However, this approach to medical therapy needs to be discussed in many cases.

In the stepwise treatment algorithm recommended by the European Glaucoma Society (EGS), pharmacological reduction of the intraocular pressure is the first step, followed by laser surgery of the trabecular meshwork and (filtering) glaucoma surgery. On the other hand, the EGS recommends that the therapeutic target for the intraocular pressure should be set as a function of the pre-existing degree of optic nerve damage, the patient's life expectancy, the rapidity of progression, and the baseline value of the intraocular pressure before treatment [6].

Over the past few years, with the introduction of newer drugs, there has been a gradual shift in the choice of medical therapy. Currently available options for medical treatment of chronic open-angle glaucoma include topical Beta adrenergic blocking agents, adrenergic drugs, miotics, carbonic anhydrase inhibitors, and prostaglandin analogues/prostamides. However, there is controversy as to the degree of reduction of IOP that can be achieved with different drugs. This controversy is fueled by the preferred citation of studies with a favorable result for certain new drugs. The results of a meta-analysis published in 2005 by van der Valk et al [7] showed that the highest reduction in IOP ranged from 33% (bimatoprost) to 17% (brinzolamide). Table 1.

Ophthalmology community has welcomed the increase in the variety of therapeutic options for our patients. However, at the same time, it has become more confused the election between the different monotherapies and the fixed or unfixed combination options.

Table 1. Overviews of the main features of some of the most prescribe antiglaucoma medications available in the market

Generic name*	% IOP Reduction from Baseline		Year of introduction	Instillation frequency	Preservative free	Wash-out time
	Peak	Trough				
Pilocarpine	25	20	1875	3-4 times daily	No	1 week
Timolol	27	26	1978	1-2 times daily	Yes	2-5 weeks
Dorzolamide	20	17	1994	2-3 times daily	Yes	1 week
Brimonidine	25	18	1996	2-3 times daily	No	1-3 weeks
Latanoprost	31	28	1996	Once daily	No	4-6 weeks
Brinzolamide	20	17	1998	2-3 times daily	No	1 week
Unoprostone	20	15	2000	2 times daily	No	4-6 weeks
Travoprost	31	29	2001	Once daily	No **	4-6 weeks
Bimatoprost (+)	33	28	2001	Once daily	No	4-6 weeks
Tafluprost	27	20	2008	Once daily	Yes	4-6 weeks

Adapted from the Guidelines of the European Glaucoma Society [6] and from van der Valk et al [7].
*Drugs are listed based on the year of introduction in the market.
** Without benzalkonium chloride.
(+) Bimatoprost 0.03%.

Additionally, it is important when selecting the medical treatment of glaucoma to understand not only the aims of therapy but also the mode of action, side effects, and contraindications of each individual medication.

There are two approaches to the medical reduction of intraocular pressure:

- Reducing the production of aqueous humor production, with the use of:
  - beta-blockers (inhibition of the beta-mediated stimulation of Na+/K+-ATPase)
  - Carbonic anhydrase inhibitors
  - Sympathomimetic drugs (activation of the alpha mediated inhibition of Na+/K+-ATPase)

- Increasing the outflow aqueous humor, with the use of:
  - Cholinergic/parasympathomimetic drugs and prostaglandin derivatives (trabecular meshwork)
  - Sympathomimetic drugs (uveoscleral outflow)
  - Prostaglandin derivatives (uveoscleral outflow)

According to the EGS guidelines, prostaglandin analogs, beta-blockers, alpha-2 agonists, and topical carbonic anhydrase inhibitors are the agents of first choice [6].

The objective of this chapter is to review the characteristics of the available antiglaucoma drugs in order to improve the management of our glaucoma patients.

2. MEDICAL TREATMENT OVERVIEW

2.1. Unilateral Trials

The monocular trials might be defined as a clinical tool designed to try to differentiate between the IOP change ascribable to the trial drug and the IOP change ascribable to unforeseen variation.

The monocular drug trial for management of glaucoma may be applied in 2 ways: (1) to assess the efficacy of a drug in the first eye treated and (2) to predict the response to a drug in the second eye treated.

Many different papers have analyzed the utility of monocular trials with conflicting results [8-11].

Despite the fact that some of these studies support the use of the monocular trials, other recommend abandoning the unilateral trial and using bilateral simultaneous trials of the same medication.

This discrepancy might stem from different study designs and methods of analysis [12].

It was recently published paper, based on the data from the Ocular Hypertension Treatment Study, which evaluated the utility of the monocular trial [13].

The relevance of this study is that it has asked an important clinical question: is the unilateral trial able to predict the trial eye`s long-term IOP reduction?

This study aimed to determine whether a monocular trial is a better assessment of medication response than testing each eye independently.

This study concluded that the monocular trial appears equivalent to testing each eye independently: However, neither method is adequate to determine medication response to topical prostaglandin analogues.

Based on the results of this study it seems that treating one eye is reasonable if only one eye needs to be treated or if there are safety concerns.

We need to start to assume that a single measurement of the IOP does not represent a valid approach to our patients.

We must accept that if we want to know whether or not a drug is effective, we must do multiples measurements of the IOP both before and after initiating therapy.

2.2. Multiple-Drug Therapy

When therapy with a single agent is inadequate to control intraocular pressure, combined treatment is indicated. Additionally, it was documented that monotherapy fails to achieve a satisfactory IOP reduction in 40-75% of glaucoma patients after more than two years of therapy [1, 4]. Adjunctive therapy may more frequently be needed in other types of glaucoma, or in advanced disease, when a greater decrease in IOP (30--40%) might be required to prevent further glaucomatous progression. With the availability of newer classes of antiglaucoma drugs the number of possible topical combinations therapies has increased enormously [14].

However, a second agent is not fully additive to the first when reductions of intraocular pressure provided by each agent separately are compared.

Nevertheless, the advantages of combine drugs are obvious. There is an additional lowering of IOP, a better 24-hours IOP profile. However, increasing the number of therapies has disadvantages as well, among them, a risk of washing of the first drug, an increase exposure to preservatives, cost, side effects, and impact of quality of life that can lead to noncompliance. Some of these disadvantages might be reduced by using fixed combinations, which will be analyzed in detail in other chapter. As a rule, drugs which belong to the same pharmacological class should not be used in combination (i.e. do not combine two different prostaglandin analogues or two topical carbonic anhydrase inhibitors (CAI)). For many years, nonselective Beta-blockers (BB) such as timolol have been the first choice in treatment for ocular hypertension (OH) and primary open-angle glaucoma (POAG). However, in the recent years, prostaglandin analogues (PGAs) have become more and more popular as first-choice drugs [15, 16] and are very often used in combination with topical BB and with topical CAI. The findings of a systematic review of the medical literature on comparative studies of fixed and unfixed adjunctive drug combinations with PGAs published in 2008 [17] suggested that adding beta-blockers and topical CAIs is more efficacious than adding alpha-adrenergic agonists. Moreover, topical CAIs have a trough IOP reduction advantage over alpha-adrenergic agonists, with a small absolute magnitude of difference, whereas the question of adequate nocturnal IOP reduction with beta-blockers remains unclear. Thus, there is some evidence that topical CAIs should be considered as the first-choice adjunctive agent to PGAs, followed by beta-blockers then alpha-adrenergic agonists.

2.3. Maximal Medical Therapy

The term maximal medical therapy is used to indicate that no further escalation of medical treatment is available or appropriate. There was a time when maximal medical therapy was interpreted to mean that every patient must be in a combination of the strongest strength of Beta-blockers, prostaglandin analogues, miotics, carbonic anhydrase inhibitors, and adrenergics before a nonmedical approach to treatment is considered. It is better to think in terms of "maximally tolerated medical therapy" that should be defined as the maximum that will be taken regularly and that will be reasonably well tolerated and effective [18]. Nowadays, the term "optimal medical therapy", which generally includes two or three medications, has replaced the concept of maximal medical therapy [19].

3. ANTIGLAUCOMA DRUGS

3.1. Adrenergic Agonist

3.1.1. Non-Selective

Epinephrine
Epinephrine was an important drug in the therapy of open-angle glaucoma. The mechanism of action is complex affecting trabecular outflow and uveoscleral outflow [20].

The increase in trabecular out flow appears to be mediated by beta-adreno receptors in the trabecular meshwork, presumably of the beta-2 subtype [21].

The minimum concentration of epinephrine required to reduce IOP is 0.12%, but greater reductions are seen at a concentration of 0.5%. However, to increase outflow a 1% concentration is required [22].

Onset of action occurs at 1 hour, with a peak effect at 4 hours. The ocular hypotensive effect may last 12 hours [23].

Long-term epinephrine therapy achieves the same degree of intraocular pressure control as timolol, although timolol appears superior in the initial year of therapy [24].

The most common adverse events of epinephrine are hyperemia, tearing, and irritation [25]. Additionally, cystoid macular edema has been reported in 10% to 20% of aphakic patients using epinephrine [26-28].

Nowadays, epinephrine might be used in patients where elevation of IOP can be deleterious for the preservation of visual function [6].

Dipivalyl-Epinephrine

Because of the use of epinephrine was limited by its bioavailability and side effects, the pro-drug form of epinephrine, dipivefrin, was synthesize.

Used in monotherapy with twice daily dosing, dipivefrin produces a 20% to 24% reduction in IOP. Dipivefrin causes less ocular discomfort than epinephrine. A common adverse effect of this drug is follicular conjunctivitis [29, 30].

The clinical indications are the same that those for epinephrine [6].

3.1.2. Alpha-2-Selective

Clonidine

Clonidine was the first relatively selective alpha-agonist identified for clinical application in ophthalmology. Concern over systemic side effects led to the development of other alpha-agonist, such as apraclonidine and brimonidine, which reduce intraocular pressure with fewer side effects.

It should be noted that, nowadays, the clinical indications of clonidine is limited for patients where elevation of IOP can be deleterious for the preservation of visual function [6].

Apraclonidine

Apraclonidine is an imidazoline derivative that differs from clonidine by the addition of an amide group. This drug lowers IOP by suppressing aqueous humor production without altering the outflow facility [31].Apraclonidine is commercially available in concentrations of 0,5% for chronic use and 1% for short term applications.

The maximal effect is observed 3 to 5 hours after dosing. At peak effect, apraclonidine 1% lowers IOP 30 to 40% from baseline and at trough 20% to 30% [32, 33].

The most troublesome side effect of chronic apraclonidine use appears to be an allergic blepharoconjunctivitis and dermatitis, similar to that seem with epinephrine and dipivefrin [33]. The most common nonocular side effect of apraclonidine is dry mouth and dry nose.

Clinical indications of apraclonidine 0.5% cover temporary chronic dosing as adjunctive treatment on maximally tolerated medical therapy where additional IOP reduction is required.

However, the addition of apraclonidine to patients already using two aqueous humor suppressing drugs may not provide additional IOP lowering effect [6].

Apraclonidine 1% is used to prevent the elevations in IOP following anterior segment laser procedures [6].

Brimonidine

Brimonidine tartrate (Alphagan; Allergan, Irvine, California, USA) is a highly selective a2-adrenergic agonist that increases uveoscleral outflow and reduces aqueous humor production [34].

A meta-analysis of randomized control trials found that brimonidine, twice daily, produced similar mean decreases in the IOP at peak compared with timolol (25%), but at trough (18%), the hypotensive effect was less than with timolol[7].

The results of recent studies showed a significant difference in the IOP lowering effect of brimonidine monotherapy between diurnal/wake and nocturnal/sleep periods [35, 36]. During the nocturnal period brimonidine showed a lack of IOP lowering efficacy [36].

On the other hand, recent experimental and animal models suggest a neuroprotective effect of brimonidine. These investigations indicate that it might have therapeutic effects if used clinically to treat optic neuropathies in humans.

However, although experimental evidence has demonstrated that brimonidine is a potential neuroprotective agent. However, to date, clinical trials have failed to translate into similar efficacy in humans.

Currently, only one study is available on brimonidine and visual function. Krupin et al [37]. This study compared the alpha2-adrenergic agonist brimonidine tartrate 0.2% to the beta-adrenergic antagonist timolol maleate 0.5% in preserving visual function in low-pressure glaucoma [37]. The results of this study suggested that the patients treated with brimonidine monotherapy were statistically less likely to have progressive visual field loss than those patients randomized to monotherapy with timolol, despite known similar IOP lowering [37].However, the most important limitation of this study is the high number of drop outs in the brimonidine group. The failure to obtain information from the dropouts limits interpretation of the results, and the unequal dropout between the groups could introduce bias if patients who dropped out were also more likely to have shown progression [37].

The most common side effects reported with brimonidine are dry mouth, conjunctival blanching, and drowsiness. Nevertheless, evaluating efficacy and safety of brimonidine 0.2%, various studies have supported its overall safety and tolerability: no clinically significant effects on mean heart rate, blood pressure or pulmonary function [38, 39].

A reformulated solution of brimonidine was released, preserved with chlorine dioxide(Purite™) rather than benzalkonium chloride (BAK), and reduced the concentration of brimonidine to 0.15%.This formulation (brimonidine 0.15% Purite), despite having 25% less active drug than brimonidine 0.2%, has comparable hypotensive efficacy, as well as having 41% lower incidence of allergic conjunctivitis [40, 41].

Brimonidine is absolutely contra-indicated in children; because of a less mature blood-brain barrier, they are susceptible to potentially serious central nervous system side effects including sleepiness, lethargy, bradycardia, hypotension, apnea and coma [42].

Brimonidine tartrate may be used as initial therapy and as adjunctive therapy as well [6].

3.2. Adrenergic Antagonist

Introduction

The Beta-adrenergic antagonists or Beta-blockers (BB) have been the most commonly used class of drugs for treating glaucoma. Because of their efficacy and minimal ocular side effects, these drugs usually were, for many years, the first-line agents for medical therapy of all types of glaucoma.

However, the initial hope of a side effect–free class of drugs has proven illusory. Although the topical side effects were few, the long-term systemic side effects of the beta-blocking agents have been shown to be many, often profound and, yet, frequently subtle.

Exacerbation of asthma and chronic obstructive pulmonary disease due to induced bronchospasm are well known side effects; therefore, these agents are usually avoided in those patients with a history of bronchospastic disorders [43].Less well known is the fact that, even in someone with no history of asthma or obstructive airway disease, topical nonselective beta-blockers can be associated with a reduction in pulmonary function [44].Bradycardia is another potential side effect, as are other forms of conduction defects. After prolonged use, depression, mood alterations, memory loss, hallucinations, decreased libido, and impotence can all occur [45].

These types of side effects are probably more common than generally acknowledged or appreciated because ophthalmologists usually don't ask about them and patients do not associate systemic side effects with topical agents. Topical beta-blockers can be associated with dry eyes and superficial punctate keratopathy [46, 47].

Finally, topical beta-blockers may have a diminished effect if the patient is already using a systemic beta-blocker [48].

The first BB evaluated for use in ophthalmology was propranolol, which lowered IOP when given intravenously [49].

Beta-blockers can be divided into two main groups: nonselective beta1-and-Beta2-adrenoreceptor antagonist, and Beta1-selective antagonist. Each of the specific agents of these two groups has individual differences in pharmacology, efficacy, tolerability, and cost. The relative beta, and beta, selectivity of various ophthalmic drugs is shown in Table 2.

Table 2.Beta adrenergic antagonists available in the market

Generic name*	Concentration (%)	Beta-1-Selective	ISA* Activity
Befunolol	0.50	No	No
Betaxolol	0.25, 0.5	Yes	No
Carteolol	0.5, 1, 2	No	yes
Levobunolol	0.25, 0.5	No	No
Metipranolol	0.1, 0.3	No	No
Pindolol	2	No	yes
Timolol	0.1, 0.25, 0.5	No	No

Adapted from the Guidelines of the European Glaucoma Society [6].
*ISA: Intrinsic sympathomimetic activity.

Timolol

The introduction of timolol in 1976 was a milestone in ocular pharmacology [50-52]. It was the first topical BB approved in the United States for the treatment of glaucoma and ocular hypertension.

Timolol decreases aqueous humor production [53] with little or no significant effect on episcleral venous pressure," outflow facility or uveoscleral flow [54]. Thus, the mechanism of the ocular hypotensive action of timolol appears to be solely a decrease in aqueous humor production.

A meta-analysis of randomized control trials found that the IOP lowering effect of timolol ranged from 27%, at peak, and 26 %, at trough [7].

It produces an ocular hypotensive effect in normal volunteers [50], in patients with ocular hypertension [55], and in those with chronic open-angle glaucoma [56].

Timolol is commercially available in 0.1%, 0.25%, and 0.5%. Concentrations higher than 0.5% provide no additional effect, indicating that this concentration is at the top of the dose-response curve [55]. Onset of IOP reduction usually occurs within 30 to 60 minutes after topical instillation. The maximal effect is after 2 hours and with chronic administration may maintain the reduction for at least 24 hours [53].

The typical administration for most patients is twice daily, although many patients can be maintained adequately with once daily administration [57].

The most common side effects were previously mentioned in the introduction.

Timolol is still commonly used as first-line choice therapy for the treatment of patients with chronic open-angle glaucoma and those with ocular hypertension.

Timolol is contraindicated in individuals with asthma, chronic obstructive pulmonary disease, and myasthenia gravis. Although it often is safely administered during pregnancy, timolol only should be used if the potential benefit justifies the potential risk to the fetus or the infant [6].

Levobunolol

Levobunolol hydrochloride is a propranolol analog with potent non-selective Beta-adrenergic antagonism. Similar to timolol, levobunolol has been reported to have no effect on uveoscleral flow, outflow facility, or episcleral venous pressure [58].

Efficacy of levobunolol is similar to timolol in side effects and IOP reduction. Numerous studies have demonstrated the drug`s long-term efficacy [59-61].

A double-mask study including 391 patients with ocular hypertension or glaucoma found sustained mean reduction in IOP of 27% over 2 years [60].

Additionally, Wandel et al. [62] evaluated the efficacy of once-daily levobunolol 0.5% and 1.0%, and timolol 0.5%. The control rate for the three treatment groups was 72%, 79%) and 64%, respectively. From a baseline intraocular pressure of 28.2 mm Hg, 26.9 mm Hg and 26.4 mm Hg, the overall decrease for the three months of the study was 7 mm Hg (29%), 6.5 mm Hg (25%) and 4.5 mm Hg (20%), respectively. The0.5% levobunolol group was statistically, different from the timolol group with respect to overall intraocular pressure.

In clinical trials levobunolol was well tolerated by most patients, with no significant difference in adverse effects compared with timolol [63].

The clinical indications for levobunolol are similar than those for timolol.

Levobunolol is contraindicated in individuals with asthma, chronic obstructive pulmonary disease, and myasthenia gravis.

Carteolol

Carteolol is a non-selective Beta-blocker, with some intrinsic sympathomimetic activity.

Structurally related to timolol, levobunolol, and betaxolol. Ocular carteolol reduces intraocular pressure in patients with open-angle glaucoma (OAG) or ocular hypertension (OH). Twice-daily administration of standard carteolol has generally similar IOP-lowering efficacy to other ocular beta-adrenoceptor antagonists such as timolol, betaxolol, and levobunolol in patients with OAG or OH. In addition, long-term treatment with carteolol has similar efficacy to timolol and betaxolol in terms of reducing IOP and maintaining visual fields in patients with newly diagnosed primary OAG (POAG). The new long-acting formulation of once-daily carteolol has equivalent efficacy to the standard formulation of carteolol administered twice daily in patients with OAG or OH. Both the standard and long-acting formulations of ocular carteolol are generally well tolerated in terms of topical adverse effects involving the eyes or systemic adverse effects involving the cardiovascular system [64].

Carteolol's efficacy and safety are similar to those of timolol. Because carteolol might have fewer deleterious effects on the lipid profile [65], some ophthalmologist may prefer it in patients with hypercholesterolemia.

Betaxolol

Betaxolol hydrochloride was introduced in the early 1980s as the first topical, cardio selective, Beta1-adrenergic antagonist for ophthalmology [66].

Betaxolol's mechanism of action is similar to that of timolol. Although there is definitive proof, betaxolol is thought to reduce aqueous humor formation through blockade of the beta-receptors of the nonpigmental cilliary epithelium [67]. Several explanations have been postulated for the ocular hypotensive effect of betaxolol: betaxolol may not be completely beta1-selective, allowing some of the drug to block the beta2-adrenoreceptors in the cilliary body; beta1-adrenoreceptoras are involved in the production of aqueous humor; or inhibition of aqueous humor is not related to beta-blockade [68].

Topical betaxolol can lower both normal and elevated intraocular pressure [66, 68].

Caldwell et al [69] found betaxolol 0.25% to be 3.0 mm Hg better than vehicle. Feghali and Kauftnant [68] found betaxolol 0.25% to be 3.7 mm Hg better than vehicle, although this difference was not statistically significant. Radius [70] found betaxolol 0.125% to be 3.9 mm Hg better than vehicle at most visits.

Allen et al [71] evaluated betaxolol and timolol in a double-masked, parallel study. They found both agents effective; however, the decrease in intraocular pressure with betaxolol, approximately 5.7 mm Hg, was statistically significantly less than with timolol, 7.4 mm Hg.

In fact most clinical trials comparing it with timolol have shown betaxolol to be statistically less effective in both lowering IOP [72, 73] and reducing aqueous flow [74].

Regarding adverse effects, although it can provoke asthma [75], several studies have shown betaxolol to be better tolerated than nonselective beta-adrenergic antagonist in patients with pulmonary disease [76-78].

Betaxolol seems to be better tolerated topically in most patients sensitive to nonselective beta-adrenergic antagonist [6].

The clinical indications for betaxolol are similar than those for timolol.

3.3. Carbonic Anhydrase Inhibitors

Introduction

Systemic carbonic anhydrase inhibitors (CAI) have been an integral part of glaucoma therapy for the past 60 years. They are among the most powerful medications for lowering IOP; unfortunately, their use is frequently accompanied by undesirable side effects which stem from the extra ocular inhibition of the enzyme carbonic anhydrase.

Carbonic anhydrase (CA) catalyzes the reversible reaction:

$$CO_2 + OH^- \ HCO_3$$

By accelerating the reversible conversion of carbon dioxide to bicarbonate, CA facilitates secretory and excretory process in several tissues.

There are at least fourteen isoenzymes of CA [79]. It has been known for some time that CA-II (previously designated as isoenzyme C) was the predominant isoenzyme found within the cilliary epithelia [80]. Patients with autosomal recessive CA-II deficiency did not show a decrease in IOP with administration of acetazolamide [81].

Carbonic anhydrase is a key enzyme in aqueous humor production. The aqueous humor flow rate in humans is approximately 2.8 μl/min during the day and decreases to about 1.2 μl/min at night. After topical application of dorzolamide or brinzolamide in healthy subjects, aqueous humor formation was reduced by 14% and 19%, respectively, during the day and by 8% and 16%, respectively, at night, which did not represent a statistically significant difference [82].

3.3.1. Topical Carbonic Anhydrase Inhibitors

Dorzolamide

In 1995 the United States Food and Drug Administration approved dorzolamide, a topically active carbonic anhydrase inhibitor (CAI), for the treatment of elevated intraocular pressure (IOP).

Dorzolamide is a heterocyclic thieno-thiopyran with sufficient lipophilicity to penetrate the eye after topical administration [83].

Dorzolamide, which is now in clinical use, was the last of the three compounds to undergo clinical testing. Due to its shorter alkyl substituent it had higher water solubility (2% at pH 6.0, 3% at pH 5.5) and less lipid solubility than either sezolamide or MK- 927. At the same time it showed higher in vitro activity against carbonic anhydrase II and IV, with an IC_{50} of 0.18 nM and 6.9 nM while it is a much weaker inhibitor of human carbonic anhydrase isoenzyme I (IC_{50} of 600 nM) [84].

The optimal concentration and frequency for dorzolamide had to be determined. A sample of 332 patients with glaucoma or ocular hypertension received dorzolamide 0.2%, 0.7%, or 2% three times daily (TID) over a period of 6 weeks. The 0.2% solution had the least hypotensive effect while the 0.7% and 2% solutions showed similar activities [85]. A 3% solution was less effective than the 2% solution [83], possibly because of increased tearing and drug wash out.

Over the different concentrations, IOP reductions ranged from 9 to 21% for twice daily (BID) and from 14 to 24% for TID administration. Three times daily administration of 2% dorzolamide induced a mean percent decrease in IOP of 18 to 22% (mean decrease 4.5-6.1 mm Hg). Over the 12-hour study period, the TID dosing regimen showed a greater IOP reduction immediately before dosing and after 10 and 12 hours [85]. However, these differences were not statistically significant. A meta-analysis of randomized control trials found that the IOP lowering effect of dorzolamide ranged from 22%, at peak, and 17 %, at trough [7].

Carbonic anhydrase inhibitors reduce IOP by lowering aqueous humor production. Partial therapeutic additivity would be expected when these drugs are used in conjunction with medications acting by different mechanisms.

The additional IOP reduction for patients receiving dorzolamide ranged from 13% to 21% [83]. O'Connor et al [86] determined the additive intraocular pressure reduction of topical dorzolamide used adjunctively with latanoprost.

When added to latanoprost, dorzolamide lowered intraocular pressure an additional 3.9 mm Hg (19.7%, P <.001).

The 2009 World Glaucoma Association consensus group [87] recognized that the topical carbonic anhydrase inhibitors (CAIs) have repeatedly shown to increase ocular blood flow and enhance blood flow regulation independent of their hypotensive effects.

The most recent comprehensive analysis on the topic of CAIs and ocular blood flow was a 2009 meta-analysis examining all published studies that investigated topical CAIs [88]. This study found consistent significant increases in numerous ocular blood flow parameters during topical CAI treatment.

The relevance of these findings, however, is critically dependent on whether preservation and/or improvement of the ocular hemodynamics contribute to visual field preservation in glaucoma, which remains insufficiently investigated.

In one four-year study [89] comparing the effects of dorzolamide 2% BID plus timolol 0.5% BID versus timolol 0.5% BID the dorzolamide plus timolol group had significantly decreased IOP, a decreased risk of visual field progression and improved retrobulbar blood flow. However, there are some important limitations in this pilot study.

Another prospective, randomized, evaluator masked parallel study that aimed to identify progression factors in POAG patients , including the effects of treatment with dorzolamide 2% or brinzolamide 1%, each added to timolol 0.5%, was recently published by Martínez and Sánchez [90].The results of this study suggested that treatment with the dorzolamide–timolol combination reduced the relative risk for progression by 48% compared with treatment with brinzolamide– timolol; p = 0.009).

However, as with the other studies on this topic several limitations should be considered when interpreting data from this research.

Side effects may be local or systemic. Although systemic CAIs exhibit rather strong systemic side effects and few local side effects, the reverse is true for dorzolamide. The following have been described during therapy with dorzolamide 2% TID. for 1 year: stinging (7%)) burning or foreign body sensation (12%)and tearing and blurring of vision (9%) [83].

In a five-year follow-up study Martinez and Sánchez-Salorio [91] found that the most frequently reported adverse event with dorzolamide was itching, which occurred in 35.7% (25/70) of patients. Additionally, this study also found that at least one adverse event was reported by 47/70 (67.1%) patients receiving dorzolamide [91].

One side effect of dorzolamide therapy that is particularly frequent (27%) and should be mentioned to patients before initiating treatment is an unusually bitter or metal-like taste.

Dorzolamide is useful in treating ocular hypertension and many types of glaucoma, including primary open-angle glaucoma, pseudo exfoliation glaucoma, [83] and pigment dispersion glaucoma.

Dorzolamide cannot be recommended for the treatment of acute angle-closure glaucoma. Repeated dorzolamide drops did not break attacks of acute angle-closure glaucoma in seven patients with IOPs equal to or higher than 50 mm Hg [83].

Brinzolamide

Brinzolamide is a topically active carbonic anhydrase inhibitor derived from a novel class of heterocyclic sulfonamides developed to lower elevated intraocular pressure. The molecular structure is similar to dorzolamide, but a side chain was added that makes brinzolamide more lipophilic than dorzolamide or acetazolamide at a physiological pH.

The optimal concentration and dosing scheme for brinzolamide was determined in two studies. Silver et al [93] reported the dose response for BID brinzolamide, 0.3%, 1%, 2%, and 3%, for two weeks in primary open-angle glaucoma patients. The maximal effect was reached at a concentration of 1%.

Brinzolamide suspension provides statistically significant IOP reductions from baseline. March and Ochner [94] reported that the IOP-lowering efficacy remained stable during a period of 18 months with a mean IOP change of -3.5 and 3.3 mm Hg at 1 and 18 months, respectively.

Sall et al. [95] compared the efficacy and safety of treatment with brinzolamide BID or TID with dorzolamide TID in patients with glaucoma and found an equivalent IOP reduction by brinzolamide (16 to 19%) TID and dorzolamide (17 to 20%) TID. Brinzolamide BID was slightly less effective but statistically and clinically equivalent to the other treatments.

As dorzolamide, brinzolamide appears to have an additional effect on IOP in patients with inadequately controlled IOP on timolol 0.5% treatment. The additional IOP reduction following brinzolamide ranged from 13 to 17 % [96].

In a prospective, randomized, evaluated-mask, and parallel study published recently by Martínez and Sánchez, [91] brinzolamide 1% when added to timolol 0.5% BID showed an IOP lowering effect similar to dorzolamide 2% added to timolol 0.5% BID.

Ishikawa and Yoshitomi[97] compared the effect of the concomitant use of brinzolamide and latanoprost on the 24-hour variation in intraocular pressure (IOP) in primary open-angle glaucoma (POAG) patients first treated with timolol and latanoprost. The results of this study suggested that when taken together, the combination of brinzolamide and latanoprost demonstrated an improved hypotensive effect in open-angle glaucoma patients compared to timolol and latanoprost during a 24-hour period [97].

As regards the side effects, brinzolamide seems to have less side effects that dorzolamide [95].

In a five-year follow-up study Martinez and Sánchez-Salorio [91] found that the most frequently reported adverse event with brinzolamide was itching, which occurred in 28.9% (22/76) of patients. Additionally, this study also found that at least one adverse event was reported by 49/76 (64.5%) patients receiving dorzolamide [91]. However, a significantly greater proportion of patients in the brinzolamide/timolol group reported blurred vision (26.3%; 20/76) as compared with the dorzolamide/timolol group (7.1%; 5/70), P = 0.002 [91].

Relatively few studies have evaluated the effect of brinzolamide upon OBF. Our findings partially disagree with those published by Kaup and colleagues [98] who reported that retrobulbar hemodynamics remained unaltered in healthy subjects treated with brinzolamide 1% BID.

The clinical indications and contraindications for brinzolamide are similar than those for dorzolamide.

3.3.2. Systemic Carbonic Anhydrase Inhibitors

Systemic carbonic anhydrase inhibitors have been an integral part of glaucoma medical therapy for the past 60 years. Their ability to lower IOP was discovered shortly after acetazolamide was marketed as an oral diuretic agent for the reduction of blood pressure [99].

Their primary mechanism of action is to reduce aqueous humor production without significantly affecting outflow facility.

The clinical indication of systemic CAIs is when topical medications are not effective or feasible. When long-term treatment with systemic CAI is needed, glaucoma surgery should be considered [6].

Acetazolamide

The clinical dose for chronic use ranges from 250 mg TID to 500 mg TID. As systemic effects are often correlated with the dose and plasma levels, it is prudent to titrate up from a sub-maximal dose. Acetazolamide decreases IOP within one hour, with a peak effect after 6 to 8 hours [100]. When given intravenously at 5 mg/kg, a decrease in pressure was noted at 2 minutes post dose, with a peak effect by 10 to 15 minutes [101]. When acetazolamide is added to treatment with topical timolol or betaxolol, pressure is reduced an additional 3 to 4 mm Hg [102].

Methazolamide

The usual dose is 50 to 100 mg BID. It is prudent to titrate up from 25 to 50 mg BID because low doses may reduce IOP with decrease adverse reactions [103].

At low dose, 25 or 50 mg BID, methazolamide decreased IOP by 2.5 to 3 mmHg compared with a 5 to 6 mm Hg reduction with 500 mg sustained-release acetazolamide BID. However, the methazolamide response was achieved with fewer adverse reactions compared with acetazolamide [103].

Dichlorphenamide

The recommended chronic dose for Dichlorphenamide is 25 to 50 mg once to three times daily. Intraocular pressure lowering effect appears comparable to other systemic CAI with similar or slightly worse tolerance [104].

Side Effects of Systemic Carbonic Anhydrase Inhibitors

Up to one half of patients are unable to tolerate the adverse effects of therapeutic systemic doses of CAI. All the available agents produce similar types of reactions, although the extent and severity vary by agent and dose [104].

The most frequent adverse effects can be grouped as a malaise complex consisting of general malaise, fatigue, weight loss, depression, and anorexia and loss of libido [105].

Additionally, patients may complain of gastrointestinal distress with nausea, epigastria burning, abdominal cramps, or diarrhea.

Paresthesias of extremities are extremely commons but usually do not lead to discontinuation of therapy by itself. Its cause is unknown.

The incidence of urolithiasis is increased approximately tenfold in patients receiving acetazolamide. The incidence also appears increased with methazolamide, but possibly to a lesser extends [105].

The most serious adverse event of systemic CAIs is the occurrence of blood dyscrasias, especially aplastic anemia.

Other side effects include hearing dysfunction, tinnitus, taste alteration, and vomiting.

Adverse effect common to all sulfonamide derivatives may occur like anaphylaxis, fever rash, Steven-Johnson syndrome, hemolytic anemia, and pancytopenia.

Because systemic CAIs have a teratogenic effect in animals [106] only to be used if the potential benefit justifies the potential risk to the fetus or the infant.

3.4. Parasympathomimetics

Ocular cholinergic agents are a group of medications used topically in the treatment of glaucoma to lower IOP.

Cholinergic drugs have been the mainstay of the medical management of most types of glaucoma since the latter half of the nineteen century.

The ocular cholinergic agents can be divided into two groups based on the site of action: Direct and Indirect.

Direct-acting drugs function directly at the neuromuscular junction of the parasympathetic nervous system to stimulate the effector muscle. Members of this group include acetylcholine hydrochloride, pilocarpine, and carbachol.

Indirect-acting parasympathomimetics, also known as anticholinesterase agents, stimulate the parasympatheticnervous system by binding the enzymes acetyl cholinesterase and butyrylcholinesterase [107].

Direct-acting parasympathomimetics are contraindicated in patients younger than 40 year-old, cataract, uveitis, and neovascular glaucoma. Indirect-acting parasympathomimetics should be used with extreme caution in patients with marked vagotonia. Furthermore, indirect-acting parasympathomimetics are contraindicated in pregnancy and nursing mothers.

Pilocarpine

Pilocarpine became available in the western countries in the 1870s, when Brazilian physician, Coutinbou, first brought it to Paris from Pernambuco, where it had been used by the natives [107].

Several German physicians explored the uses of the drug and noticed its ocular effects, including IOP reduction [108].

Pilocarpine acts at the parasympathetic muscarinic receptor site, as does the physiological mediator, acetylcholine. Contraction of the cilliary muscle produces tension on the scleral spur, to which the cilliary muscle is attached. This posterior stretching of the scleral spur is thought to produce traction on the trabecular meshwork, pulling it open and facilitating aqueous humor outflow and lowering of IOP.

Although a wide range of concentrations of pilocarpine is available, the 1 to 4% solutions are most commonly used. Drance and Nash [109] showed that pilocarpine concentrations greater than 4% do not generally augment the ocular hypotensive effect.

Pilocarpine shows an additive hypotensive effect when used in conjunction with other agents in the therapy of open-angle glaucoma.

The most common side effects of pilocarpine are reduced vision in low illumination secondary to pupillary miosis, induced myopia, and supraorbital and temporal headaches attributable to stimulation of the cilliary muscle.

Systemic side effects result from activation of muscarinic receptor and smooth muscle of the gastrointestinal tract, pulmonary system, urinary tract, and sweat gland with administration of large doses of pilocarpine and results in nausea, vomiting, diarrhea, sweating, bronchial spasm, slowing of the heart.

Carbachol

Like pilocarpine charbacol reduces intraocular pressure by increasing aqueous outflow. The drug typically is given three times daily.

Intraocular charbacol was developed for use in intraocular surgery to produce prolonged miosis. Intraocular charbacol not only produces prolonged miosis but also results in a significant reduction in postoperative IOP after cataract surgery [110].

Charbacol has most of the same local side effects as the other parasympathomimetics, although they are somewhat more severe and more common than those caused by pilocarpine. Systemic side effects are encountered somewhat more often with the use of charbacol than with pilocarpine, particularly increased salivation, diarrhea, gastric secretion, bradycardia, and bronchial constriction. Because of its side effects, charbacol is relatively contraindicated in patients with severe respiratory, cardiovascular or gastrointestinal tract disease.

3.5. Prostaglandin Analogues and Prostamides

Prostaglandin (PG) analogues are a novel class of intraocular-lowering medications used primarily for the treatment of glaucoma.

Their ability to effectively reduce intraocular pressure with once-per-day dosing, their comparable ocular tolerability with timolol, and their general lack of systemic side effects have made them the mainstay of pharmacological therapy for glaucoma and ocular hypertension in most parts of the world.

Probably, the most attractive feature of PG analogs is their ability to significantly reduce IOP with only one-daily administration in patients with glaucoma or ocular hypertension. In fact, their IOP-lowering effect is decreased if used more than once daily.

Today, the PG analogs used clinically for their IOP-lowering activity are all derivatives of naturally occurring PGF2a. Slight differences exist in their chemical structures, including the saturation of the double bond between the carbon-13 and carbon-14 positions of latanoprost.

These drugs reduce IOP by stimulation of aqueous humor drainage primarily through the uveoscleral outflow pathway but significant effects on trabecular outflow facility also have been reported [111, 112].

To date, three prostaglandin derivatives (latanoprost, travoprost, and bimatoprost) have been marketed across the world. In addition, unoprostone is prescribed in Japan and in 2008 tafluprost was marketed in some European countries and in Japan.

Ocular side effects with a well-established cause and- effect relationship to topical PGA therapy include conjunctival hyperemia, eyelash changes, induced iris darkening, and periocular skin pigmentation.

Other potential side effects are significantly less common, but have more serious sight-threatening consequences. These include iris cysts, cystoid macular edema, anterior uveitis, and reactivation of herpes simplex keratitis. Most of the reported experience with both the common and less common side effects has been associated with latanoprost, presumably because it was the first PGA to be studied. Aside from less conjunctival hyperemia with latanoprost, however, there is no evidence that any of the commercially available PGAs differ significantly with regard to side effects, and clinicians must be alert to all of these reported side effects when prescribing any PGA to their glaucoma patients [113].

Latanoprost

In 1996, Pharmacia marketed latanoprost (Xalatan; now marketed by Pfizer Inc., New York, NY), which was dosed once daily. Latanoprost the first prostaglandin to become commercially available is used once daily and produces a 28 to 31% reduction in IOP [7].

All the reported studies clearly indicate that once daily application of latanoprost at the concentration of 0.005% is sufficient to lower IOP at statistically and clinically significant levels. This conclusion has been substantiated in three large Phase 3 clinical studies [113].

Interestingly, in a large, long-term, Phase 3 clinical trial using a cross-over design, 0.005% latanoprost applied in the evening was found to be more effective in reducing diurnal IOP than morning application of the same concentration [114].

A pooled data analysis (pooling of data from independent multiple trials) of three phase III clinical trials conducted in Scandinavia, the UK, and the United States showed that latanoprost reduced the mean diurnal IOP by 7.7 (31%, SEM 0.1) mm Hg from an overall untreated mean diurnal IOP of 24.8 mm Hg (SEM 0.1) after 6 months of double-masked treatment [115].

Additionally, a pooled data analysis of three randomized, double-masked, multicenter, parallel group, 6-month studies conducted in the United States, United Kingdom, and Scandinavia compared the efficacy and safety of latanoprost and timolol suggested that latanoprost provides superior IOP reduction compared with timolol in patients with OH [116].

Alm et al. [117] evaluated the 5-year safety and efficacy of adjunctive 0.005% latanoprost once daily. The study was conducted in Patients with primary open-angle or exfoliation glaucoma that completed a 3-year, open-label; uncontrolled, prospective trial could enter a 2-year extension phase. The results of this study found that the overall mean intraocular pressure reduction from baseline of 25% was sustained with no need for change in intraocular pressure-lowering treatment in 70% of the eyes.

The majority of the studies that compared the efficacy and safety of latanoprost and travoprost [118] or of latanoprost and bimatoprost [119, 120] have shown no clinically significant differences in the IOP-lowering ability of these medications at 8 AM, the time of peak effect, and differences at other time points may have been confounded by baseline differences.

Parrish et al [121] in a 12-week, randomized, parallel-group, masked-evaluator study conducted at 45 sites in the United States compared the efficacy and safety of once daily administration of latanoprost 0.005%, bimatoprost 0.03%, and travoprost 0.004% ophthalmic solutions. The results of this study concluded that latanoprost, bimatoprost, and travoprost are equally potent IOP-lowering treatments that are generally well tolerated systemically. Significantly fewer patients reported symptoms of ocular hyperemia with latanoprost treatment [121].

Additionally most studies with these types of drugs have included Caucasian patients. However, some reports have suggested that there is a difference in response between patients of white and African racial heritage [122, 123].

Birt et al. [124] compared the effectiveness and safety of latanoprost, travoprost, and bimatoprostin people from various ethnic heritages.

No differences in effect between the drugs or between members of different racial groups were detected, although the study sample size was too small to be certain to detect differences, if they existed [124].

Latanoprost was shown to be additive to the IOP-lowering effects of some other currently used glaucoma drugs in ocular hypertensive and primary open-angle glaucoma patients.

O'Connor et al evaluated all three classes of additive therapy in 73 eyes with pressures inadequately controlled by latanoprost monotherapy [86]. In that retrospective review, adjunctive therapy with dorzolamide dosed twice or three times daily provided a statistically greater IOP reduction than the addition of beta-blockers or brimonidine [86].

Otherwise, in two combined multi-center trials, Zabriskie and associates found that a combination of brimonidine tartrate and latanoprost provided superior IOP control compared to the dorzolamide/timolol fixed combination at the morning peak measurement [125].

Aside from less conjunctival hyperemia with latanoprost, however, there is no evidence that any of the commercially available PGAs differ significantly with regard to side effects.

An interesting finding was the possible effect of the prostaglandin analogs on the central corneal thickness (CCT). Hatanaka et al [126] evaluated the influence of prostaglandin analogs and prostamides on CCT. The results of this study suggested that topical therapy with prostaglandin analogs and bimatoprost is associated with CCT reduction over a period of at least 8 weeks.

Travoprost

Travoprost (Travatan™ [Alcon, Ft Worth, TX]), a PGF2a analog, is an isopropyl ester of the (+) enantiomer of fluprostenol. Chemically it has the name isopropyl (Z)-7-[1R, 2R, 3R, 5S) -3, 5- dihydroxy -2- [(1E, 3R)-3- hydroxyl -4-[(α, α ,α-tri fluoro-m-tolyl) oxy]-1-butenyl) cyclopentyl]-5-heptenoate.

It is structurally similar to other prostaglandin F2a analogs such as latanoprost [127, 128].

Travoprost increased uveoscleral outflow in monkeys [129] and marginally increased it in ocular hypertensive patients as well [130].

The results of a randomized, prospective, active-control (timolol), parallel group study found that travoprost 0.004% lowered IOP more than timolol in 11 of 15 measurement time points, from 0.7 to 1.4mm Hg. Change from baseline demonstrated a 30– 33% decrease for travoprost compared with a 25–29% decrease for timolol [131].

Additionally, a randomized, prospective, active-control (timolol), parallel group, and 12-months study included 801 patients with open-angle, exfoliation, pigmentary glaucoma or ocular hypertension in a four group 1:1:1:1 design [118].

Groups included the following: travoprost 0.0015%, once-daily, n= 205; travoprost 0.004%, once-daily, n=200; latanoprost 0.005%, once-daily, n=196; and timolol 0.5%, twice-daily, n =200.

Compared with baseline, travoprost and timolol significantly reduced IOP by 7.1 mm Hg (28%) and 5.9 mm Hg (23%), respectively. At every study time point, the IOP reduction was greater for travoprost than for timolol. Combining the 18 study measurements, the average difference in IOP between timolol and travoprost was 1.4 mm Hg. It can be concluded that travoprost 0.004% was more effective at lowering IOP than timolol [118].

Regarding latanoprost, from an average baseline IOP of 25.5 and 25.7 mm Hg for travoprost and latanoprost, respectively, mean IOP was reduced to the range of 17.5 to 19.7 mm Hg for travoprost and 17.9 to 19.5 mm Hg for latanoprost. This equates to an average decrease from baseline of 7.1 mm Hg (28%) and 7.0 mm Hg, (27%), respectively ($p > 0.05$). The overall results demonstrated that travoprost 0.004% lowered IOP equally as well as latanoprost 0.005%.

In another study, Cantor et al compared the efficiency of travoprost and bimatoprost treatment in 157 patients over six months at different time points. The mean IOP reductions with travoprost and bimatoprost were, respectively, 5.7 versus 7.1 mmHg at 9 am ($P = 0.014$), 5.2 versus 5.9 mmHg at 1 pm ($P = 0.213$), and 4.5 versus 5.3 mmHg at 4 pm ($P = 0.207$). IOP reductions $\geq 20\%$ and $\geq 30\%$ were achieved by statistically similar proportions of patients as revealed by responder analysis, and both groups presented statistically equivalent investigator-determined clinical success which was based on drug tolerability and achievement of target IOP [132].

Orzalesi et al [133] compared 24-hours IOP reduction by latanoprost 0.005%, travoprost 0.004%, and bimatoprost 0.03% in patients with POAG or ocular hypertension in a prospective, randomized, double-masked, and cross-over study. The results of this study seemed to indicate that the 3 prostaglandin analogs were effective in reducing IOP in POAG and ocular hypertensive patients throughout the circadian cycle [133].

On the other hand, a meta-analysis of 24-hour IOP studies published by Stewart et al [134] found that travoprost showed a greater reduction as compared with latanoprost [133].

As regards side effects, conjunctival hyperemia seems to be greater with travoprost than with latanoprost [121, 123, 135].

As latanoprost, travoprost was shown to be additive to the IOP-lowering effects of some other currently used glaucoma drugs in ocular hypertensive and primary open-angle glaucoma patients.

The effects of adding topical carbonic anhydrase inhibitors or topical alpha-agonists to PGAs remain little explored.

Felmand et al in a prospective, randomized, double-masked, and multicenter clinical trial found that the combination of travoprost and brinzolamide was significantly more efficacious than the combination of travoprost and brimonidine in lowering IOP [136].The addition of brinzolamide to travoprost results in IOP reductions of 13--23% (2.7-4.2 mm Hg) [136, 137].

Bimatoprost

Bimatoprost (Lumigan™ [Allergan, Inc, Irvine CA])(Z)-7-[(1R,2R,3R,5S)- 3,5-dihydroxy-2-[(1E,3S)-3-hydroxy-5-phenyl-1-pentenyl] cyclopentyl]-5-N-ethylheptenamide, has a chemical structure similar to PGF 2α analogs, although it reportedly is not a PG and does not act on prostanoid receptors [138].

Bimatoprost has been commercially available since March 2001. It has been classified as a prostamides, which is a structural analogue related to prostaglandin F2α. It has been hypothesized that the bimatoprost acts on novel receptors that are heterodimers with the wild-type prostaglandin F receptor and a newly identified splice variant of the prostaglandin F receptor. Recently, a selective prostamides antagonist has been reported [139].

The ocular hypotensive mechanism of action of bimatoprost was reported in a clinical study of 25 ocular normotensive volunteers [140].

Compared with the vehicle-treated eyes, the bimatoprost treated eyes had a 20% reduction in IOP, 13% increase in aqueous humor flow, and 26% increase in outflow facility as measured by Schiötz tonography [140].

The outflow facility increase (or outflow resistance decrease) was insufficient to account for the entire IOP reduction, suggesting that either uveoscleral outflow (pressure insensitive outflow) was increased or episcleral venous pressure (extra ocular recipient pressure) was decreased.

The preponderance of evidence indicates that bimatoprost 0.03% once daily in the evening is more effective than timolol 0.5% twice daily at lowering IOP [135].

Additionally, Brandt et al found that once-daily bimatoprost reduced IOP an average of 0.9 mm Hg more than twice-daily bimatoprost.

Parrish et al compared three PGAs head-to-head in a randomized, 12-week prospective trial including 410 subjects. This group reported no differences in mean IOP reduction between travoprost (8.0 mmHg), latanoprost (8.7 mmHg), and bimatoprost (8.6 mmHg, P = 0.128) [121].

However, Faridi et al in a prospective randomized single (investigator) masked comparative clinical trial that evaluated the efficacy and tolerance of three prostaglandin analogues, bimatoprost, latanoprost and travoprost in patients with previously untreated open-angle glaucoma and ocular hypertension; reported that after 2 months of treatment, there was a significant difference between the three treatment groups (P = 0.013) with bimatoprost achieving a greater reduction in IOP than the other two drops. However, at 6 months, the difference was not statistically significant (P = 0.13) [142].

Bimatoprost 0.01% is a new formulation that was developed with the goal of creating a formulation of bimatoprost that would maintain the IOP-lowering efficacy achieved with bimatoprost 0.03% and have an improved overall safety profile, particularly improved ocular surface tolerability. The strategy was to reduce the concentration of bimatoprost and increase the concentration of benzalkonium chloride (BAK), a commonly used preservative that also can increase the corneal penetration.

In a Prospective, randomized, double-masked, multicenter clinical trial Katz et al evaluated the IOP-lowering efficacy and safety of ophthalmic formulations of bimatoprost 0.01% and 0.0125% compared with bimatoprost 0.03%.

The results of this study suggested that bimatoprost 0.01% was equivalent to bimatoprost 0.03% in lowering IOP throughout 12 months of treatment and demonstrated improved tolerability, including less frequent and severe conjunctival hyperemia. Bimatoprost 0.01% showed a better benefit-to-risk ratio than bimatoprost 0.0125% [143].

As regards side effects, several studies have demonstrated that the frequency of conjunctival hyperemia observed with bimatoprost 0.03% is about double that seen with latanoprost [121, 144,145].

In one comparative trial, the reported incidence of acquired skin pigmentation was 1.5% for latanoprost and 2.9% for bimatoprost and travoprost [121].Nevertheless, there is no evidence that this side effect occurs more often with bimatoprost than with the other PG analogs.

Additionally, the overall incidence of treatment-related adverse events was lower in the bimatoprost 0.01% group (38.4%) than in the bimatoprost 0.03% group (50.8%), and thedifference between groups was statistically significant (P=0.016) [143].

Tafluprost

Tafluprost, isopropyl (5Z)-7-((1R,2R,3R,5S)-2-((1E)-3,3-difluoro-4-phenoxybut-1-enyl) -3,5-dihydroxycyclopentyl) hept-5-enoate, is a newly synthesized prostaglandin PG (F2α) analogue under development as an ocular hypotensive drug. It is a pro-drug ester that facilitates corneal penetration and allows delivery of the active carboxylic acid form to the aqueous humor.

The IOP-lowering activity of tafluprost has been demonstrated both in ocular normotensive monkeys and in laser-induced ocular hypertensive monkeys [147]. In the former the maximal IOP reductions achieved with a single dose of tafluprost (0.00002 to 0.0025%) were dose-dependent, with statistical significance being reached at doses of 0.0005 and 0·0025%, and the potency of tafluprost at 0·0005% was almost equal to that of latanoprost at 0·005%. When normotensive monkeys received repeated doses of tafluprost (0.0015%, 0.0025%, or 0.005%) once daily for 5 days, this drug exhibited IOP-lowering effects not only on the first day, but also on the third and fifth days of administration, without an attenuation of efficacy over time [147].

It is presently available in two formulations, i.e., with benzalkonium chloride and preservative-free in Europe, both in 0.0015% (15 μg/mL) concentrations [148].

Clinical studies on tafluprost have been carried out both in Western countries [149-152] and in Japan, in each case using preservative containing tafluprost preparations.

Of the three phase III clinical studies conducted in Japan, one was designed as a non-inferiority study aimed at comparing the efficacy of tafluprost with that of latanoprost. In that study – a randomized, single-blind comparative study involving 109 patients with primary open angle glaucoma or ocular hypertension (reference drug: latanoprost ophthalmic solution) – the magnitude of the IOP reduction in the tafluprost and latanoprost treatment group after 4 week administration was 6.6 ± 2.5 mmHg (27.6 ± 9.6%) and 6.2 ± 2.5 mmHg (25.9 ± 9.7%), respectively [153].

Uusitalo et al [152] compared the long-term efficacy and safety of tafluprost 0.0015% with latanoprost 0.005% eye drops in patients with open-angle glaucoma or ocular hypertension. The results of this study suggested that both treatments had a substantial IOP-lowering effect which persisted throughout the study (-7.1 mmHg for tafluprost and -7.7 mmHg for latanoprost at 24 months). Although the IOP-lowering effect during the study was slightly larger with latanoprost, this difference was clinically small [152].

Additionally, Schnober et al. [154] in a randomized, double-masked, active-controlled, crossover design trial compared the diurnal intraocular pressure (IOP)-lowering efficacy and safety of travoprost 0.004% and tafluprost 0.0015% administered to patients with primary open-angle glaucoma or ocular hypertension. In this crossover study of patients with primary open-angle glaucoma or ocular hypertension, both travoprost and tafluprost demonstrated excellent IOP control, showing a mean 7.6 mmHg IOP reduction for travoprost and a mean 7.1 mmHg IOP reduction from baseline for tafluprost. Based on the results of this study, the 12-hour mean diurnal IOP was significantly lower with travoprost therapy than with tafluprost therapy ($P = 0.01$), and a significantly lower IOP was also reported for travoprost at five of the seven individual time points ($P < 0.05$).

Benzalkonium chloride is thought to be an ocular penetration enhancer for topically administered drugs, because it increases the corneal permeability of pharmacologic agents. Pellinen and Lokkila evaluated corneal penetration of preserved and preservative-free tafluprost 0.0015% into rabbit aqueous humor after topical application. They noticed that there were no significant between-group differences in mean concentrations of tafluprost acid in the aqueous humor. They concluded that BAK at the concentration used in the tafluprost formulations did not affect corneal penetration of this drug into rabbit aqueous humor [155].

In a Phase I study evaluating the pharmacokinetics and efficacy of preserved and preservative-free tafluprost, Uusitalo et al did not observe any significant differences in pharmacokinetic parameters between the formulations, after either single or repeated dosing [156].

Ocular hyperemia occurred with the same frequency in both groups, but was predominantly of moderate severity in eyes treated with preserved tafluprost, and of mild severity in those treated with the preservative-free formulation [156]. The safety of preserved and preservative-free tafluprost was also assessed in a Phase III study [157]. In contrast with the findings of Uusitalo et al [156] it was shown that conjunctival hyperemia was reported more often by people using preservative-free tafluprost [157]. The aforementioned studies showed that IOP reduction obtained by preservative-free tafluprost is equivalent to that achieved by the preserved formulation.

Based on the results of the published studies it seems that tafluprost has a similar safety profile than the other PG analogs.

3.6. Osmotics

Systemically administered hyperosmotic agents are effective as a short-term or emergency treatment of elevated IOP. They are useful in acute conditions such as angle-closure glaucoma and in the initial management of some open-angle glaucomas with extremely high IOP (i.e. traumatic glaucoma).

The effectiveness and duration of action of a particular hyperosmotic agent are dependent on the magnitude and duration of the induced blood-ocular osmotic gradient. Factors that influence osmotic gradient include the following:

- The dose and rate at which the drug is administered.
- The rate at which the drug is cleared from the systemic circulation

- The distribution of the drug in body fluids
- The rate of penetration and the extent to which the drug enters the eye

Hyperosmotic agents may be divided in oral and intravenous agents (Table 4).

Table 3.Parasympathomimetics available in the market

Generic name*	Concentration (%)	Type
Aceclidine	2	Direct-acting
Acetylcholine	1	Direct-acting
Carbachol	0.75, 1.5, 2.25, 3	Direct-acting
Pilocarpine	0.5, 1, 2, 3, 4	Direct-acting
Demecarium bromide	0.125, 0.25	Indirect-acting
Ecothiophate iodide	0.03, 0.25	Indirect-acting
Diisopropylfluorophophate	0.025	Indirect-acting
(DFP)-isofluorophate	0.1	Indirect-acting

Adapted from the Guidelines of the European Glaucoma Society (6) and Nardin& Zimmerman [107].

Table 4.Hyperosmotic agents available in the market

Generic name*	Dosage (g/kg)	Route of administration	Distribution	Ocular penetration
Alcohol	0.8 to 1.5	Oral	Total body water	Good
Glycerol	1 to 1.5	Oral	Extracellular	Poor
Isosorbide	1 to 1.5	Oral	Total body water	Good
Mannitol	1 to 1.5	Intravenous	Extracellular	Very poor
Urea	0.5 to 2	Intravenous	Total body water	Good

Drugs are listed in alphabetical order.

Table 5.Commercially available fixed combinations in the market

Generic name*	Combined with Beta-blocker	Brand name	Instillation Frequency
Bimatoprost 0.03%	Timolol 0.5%	Ganfort	Once daily
Brimonidine 0.2%	Timolol 0.5%	Combigan	Twice daily
Brimonidine 0.2% + dorzolamide 2%	Timolol 0.5%	KrytantecOfteno	Twice daily
Brinzolamide 1%	Timolol 0.5%	Azarga	Twice daily
Dorzolamide 2%	Timolol 0.5%	Cosopt	Twice daily
Latanoprost 0.005%	Timolol 0.5%	Xalacom	Once daily
Pilocarpine 2%	Carteolol 2%	Carpilo	Twice daily
	Metipranolol 0.1%	Ripix, Normoglaucon	Twice daily
	Timolol 0.5%	Fotil	Twice daily
Pilocarpine 4%	Timolol 0.5%	Fotil forte	Twice daily
Travoprost 0.0004%	Timolol 0.5%	DouTrav	Once daily

Drugs are listed in alphabetical order.
Adapted from the Guidelines of the European Glaucoma Society [6].

The side effects associated with hyperosmotic agents range from mild to potentially fatal. Special caution is advised in the elderly and in all patients with cardiac, renal, or hepatic disease [146].

The most common side effects are headache and back pain. Additionally, hyperosmotic agents must be used with caution in patients with renal failure.

3.7. Fixed-Combination Drugs Preparations

The most commonly used classes of IOP-lowering medications are the prostaglandin analogs, beta-adrenergic receptor antagonists (beta-blockers), alpha adrenergic receptor agonists (alpha agonists), and carbonic anhydrase inhibitors.

For many patients, a single medication is insufficient to reduce IOP to the target pressure, and the treatment regimen includes 2, 3, or more medications from different classes.

In recent years the number and use of fixed combinations of IOP-lowering medications for treatment in glaucoma and ocular hypertension has grown substantially. These fixed combinations contain 2,or in one case 3, medications in a single bottle and offer several advantages over concomitant use of the medications from separate bottles. Most important is the increase in patient convenience that results from the use of fewer bottles and eye drops of medication and sometimes from dosing fewer times each day. The improved convenience of a regimen containing a fixed combination rather than 2 separate medications is likely to lead to better adherence. Although few, if any, studies have directly evaluated adherence to IOP-lowering fixed combinations compared with the component medications used separately, there is evidence that adherence in glaucoma is better when regimens are simple rather than complex [158].

Because there is no possibility of a washout effect and no need to wait between instillation of the separate individual medications, both efficacy and adherence may be enhanced when a fixed combination is used rather than the separate component medications. Use of a fixed combination may also represent a safety improvement, because the patient's overall daily exposure to preservative may be decreased. Finally, there is potential cost savings associated with the use of fixed combinations [158].

However, we need to be cautious, as all these fixed combinations eye drops contain a Beta-blocker, it is mandatory to exclude contraindications to Beta-blockers when prescribing these fixed combination drugs.

An important disadvantage that should be highlighted is that it is not possible to change the drug concentration or dosing schedule for one component medication independently of the other when using a fixed combination.

The efficacy and safety of fixed combinations relative to their active components must be evaluated to obtain regulatory drug approval. For drug approval by the FDA, a fixed combination must have better efficacy than each of the component medications used as monotherapy. The efficacy and safety findings from comparison studies of fixed combinations and their component are summarized in Table 5.

3.7.1. Adrenergic Antagonist and Adrenergic Agonist

The fixed combination of brimonidine and timolol (BTFC) (Combigan™ [Allergan, Inc., Irvine CA]) combines two commonly used classes of IOP-lowering drugs are the Beta-adrenergic antagonists (Beta-blockers) and the Alfa-adrenergic agonists.

BTFC has shown to provide sustained IOP lowering superior to monotherapy with either thrice-daily brimonidine or twice-daily timolol.

A study reported by Sherwood et al [159] compared fixed-combination brimonidine 2%/timolol 0.5% with its component medications used separately as monotherapy. In this 12-month, randomized, double-masked study, 1159 patients with glaucoma or ocular hypertension were washed out of any previous IOP-lowering medication and randomized to treatment with BTFC BID, brimonidine 2% TID, or timolol 0.5% bid. Throughout 12 months of treatment, twice-daily BTFC was significantly more effective than either twice-daily timolol or thrice-daily brimonidine in reducing IOP. Mean IOP reductions from baseline were significantly greater with BTFC compared with timolol at all measurements ($P \leq 0.002$) and compared with brimonidine at all measurements except those at 5 PM, after the afternoon dose of brimonidine monotherapy ($P < 0.001$). As might be expected due to the addition of a second drug, the fixed combination was less well tolerated than timolol monotherapy. Interestingly, however, BTFC demonstrated an improved safety profile compared with brimonidine monotherapy [159].

As compared with the concomitant use of its components, BTFC is as safe and effective as concomitant treatment with the individual components [160].

A more recent randomized controlled trial [161] has evaluated the 24-hour IOP control of BTFC versus the combination of its individual components, each dosed twice daily, in patients with POAG or OH. Both BTFC and the unfixed components showed a significant IOP reduction from untreated baseline ($p < 0.0001$). The two treatment groups were statistically equal when compared directly, for each individual time point and for the 24-hour IOP curve ($p > 0.05$).

Many different studies have compared the efficacy and safety of the fixed combinations of brimonidine/timolol and dorzolamide/timolol (DTFC).

In a 2-month, open-label, surveillance study (CEED II) of fixed brimonidine/timolol use in 2133 patients at 123 centers in Canada, patients switched from DTFC to BTFC achieved average additional IOP lowering of 2.2 to 2.6 mmHg [162].Open-label drug replacement studies do not provide strong evidence of comparative drug efficacy, but the safety and tolerability findings of the study may be more informative. On a questionnaire given in the study, patients reported less burning, stinging, and metallic taste after switching from DTFC to BTFC, suggesting that fixed brimonidine/timolol may be better tolerated than fixed dorzolamide/timolol [162].

Similar results were found in a prospective, randomized, double-masked, crossover study [163]. This study found that reductions from baseline in mean diurnal IOP and morning IOP were greater with BTFC than with DTFC (difference: 0.95 mmHg, 95% CI 0.10-1.80, p = 0.03) [163].

Conversely, in a randomized, investigator-masked, crossover study comparing DTFC and BTFC in 30 patients, there were no statistically significant differences in efficacy after 4 weeks of treatment [164].

BTFC is indicated for the reduction of IOP in patients with POAG or OH who are insufficiently responsive to topical β-blockers. The recommended dosage is 1 drop into the affected eye twice daily.

Contraindications to BTFC include hypersensitivity to the individual components, monoamine oxidase inhibitor use, bronchospasm, bronchial asthma, severe chronic obstructive pulmonary disease, sinus bradycardia, second or third degree atrioventricular block, or overt cardiac failure or cardiogenic shock.

3.7.2. Adrenergic Antagonist and Parasympathomimetics

Pilocarpine has been used for glaucoma therapy for decades and frequently is used as "add on" therapy. Miotic treatment causes contraction of the cilliary muscle, which pulls on the scleral spur and reduces the resistance in the trabecular meshwork. This increases aqueous humor outflow through the pressure-dependent pathway and thus reduces IOP [165]. Studies of a fixed combination of timolol and pilocarpine found the combination to be more efficacious than either drug alone [166, 167].

In a randomized, double-blind, parallel-group study Demailly et al. found that the fixed combination of pilocarpine/timolol (PTFC) significantly reduced IOP in POAG patients with elevated IOP [168].

Kaluzny et al. compared the efficacy and safety of timolol maleate/dorzolamide fixed combination (DTFC) versus timolol maleate/pilocarpine fixed combination (TPFC), each given twice daily, in primary open-angle glaucoma or ocular hypertensive patients. This study suggested that TPFC can provide at least a similar efficacious reduction in IOP as DTFC in patients with primary open-angle glaucoma or ocular hypertension [169].

Recently Kaluzny and Col compared the safety and effect on intraocular pressure of latanoprost given every evening versus pilocarpine/timolol maleate fixed combination given twice daily in patients with primary open-angle glaucoma or ocular hypertension. This study concluded that Both PTFC and latanoprost are efficacious in reducing diurnal IOP in POAG or OH. However, PTFC may be more effective in the late morning and may have a greater incidence of mild ocular side-effects [170].

Since compliance with a pilocarpine regimen has been shown to be poor, with patients administering a mean of only 76% of the prescribed doses and 30% of patients compressing their doses into 12 hours of the day [171] it is likely that the use of a timolol pilocarpine combination twice daily might achieve better control and improved compliance in patients with glaucoma.

3.7.3. Adrenergic Antagonist and Prostaglandins

3.7.3.1. Fixed Combination of Latanoprost/Timolol

The first fixed combination of a prostaglandin analog and timolol to be developed was fixed-combination latanoprost 0.005%/timolol 0.5% (LTFC) (Xalacom®, Pharmacia, Kalamazoo, MI, and Pfizer, New York, NY).To date, none of the fixed combinations of a prostaglandin analog and timolol have received FDA approval for use in the United States. This fixed combination formulation was approved in Europe during the summer of 2001.

In a 6-month, randomized, double-masked study reported by Higginbotham et al. [172] of LTFC versus its component medications used as monotherapy, 418 patients run-in for 2 to 4 weeks on timolol BID were switched to LTFC once daily (QD) in the morning, latanoprost QD in the evening, or timolol BID. After 6 months, the mean change from baseline diurnal IOP was only approximately 1 mmHg larger in the LTFC group than in the latanoprost group. Similar results were reported by Pfeiffer and the German Latanoprost Fixed Combination Study Group [173]. This study compared the efficacy of a fixed combination of 0.5% timolol and 0.005% latanoprost to the individual monotherapies, latanoprost 0.005%, dosed in the morning, and timolol 0.5% BID.

LTFC reduced diurnal IOP by 1.2 mmHg more than latanoprost monotherapy and 1.9 mmHg more than timolol monotherapy. In both studies, LTFC lowered IOP substantially more than timolol alone. The differences in IOP lowering between FCLT and latanoprost alone were also statistically significant, but latanoprost monotherapy was nearly as effective as LTFC.

In a 12-week, randomized, double-masked, parallel-group study Higginbotham et al. assessed the efficacy and safety of fixed-combination latanoprost-timolol vs. latanoprost or timolol monotherapy. The results of this study showed that LTFC was statistically superior to latanoprost at 7 of 9 time points and at all 9 time points when compared with timolol. In addition, FCLT was associated with greater percentage reductions in diurnal IOP levels and a greater likelihood of achieving lower mean diurnal IOP levels. Diurnal IOP reductions of 30% or more from baseline to week 12 were achieved by 73.5%, 57.5%, and 32.8% of those treated with LTFC, latanoprost, and timolol, respectively (P = .007 for LTFC vs. timolol; P < .001 for LTFC vs. latanoprost) [174].

Additionally, a randomized, double-masked, crossover study in 195 patients showed that LTFC QD in the morning does not lower IOP as effectively as concomitant treatment with latanoprost QD in the evening and timolol BID [175]. However, a subsequent 12-week, randomized, double-masked, parallel-group study in 517 patients demonstrated that LTFC QD in the evening is as effective in lowering IOP as concomitant treatment with latanoprost QD in the evening and timolol BID [176].

The efficacy and safety of fixed combinations of latanoprost/timolol and dorzolamide/timolol in open-angle glaucoma or ocular hypertension was assessed in a prospective, randomized, evaluator-masked, multicenter, and controlled clinical trial [177]. The results of this study suggested that neither fixed combination is inferior to the other. However, a significantly greater percentage of subjects treated with FC latanoprost/timolol achieved IOP levels<or=16 and <or=15 mm Hg (P<or=0.01) [177].

Martinez et al reported that there were no statistical significant differences in the IOP lowering effect between LTFC and DTFC [178].

Additionally, the long-term effect of the DTFC and LTFC fixed combinations on intraocular pressure IOP and visual field defects over time in naïve primary open-angle glaucoma patients was assessed [179]. The results of this study suggested that the IOP lowering effect of both treatments was significant and equivalent. Nevertheless, that glaucomatous progression rate was significantly lower in the DTFC treatment group [179].

Finally, it was recently published a study that aimed to evaluate the long-term efficacy and safety of 3 commercially available fixed combinations of prostaglandin analogs or a prostamide with timolol maleate in patients with primary open angle glaucoma or ocular hypertension [180]. This study concluded that all 3 combinations are effective at lowering IOP but at 12 months latanoprost/timolol and bimatoprost/timolol (BiTFC) fixed combinations were found to be more effective than travoprost/timolol fixed combination. Treatments were well tolerated after 12 months but LTFC showed less hyperemia than BiTFC throughout the study (P < 0.05) [180].

3.7.3.2. Fixed Combination of Travoprost/Timolol

The prostaglandin analog travoprost has been combined with timolol in fixed-combination travoprost 0.004%/timolol 0.5% (TTFC) (DuoTrav®; Alcon Laboratories, Inc.).

The fixed combination of travoprost/timolol (TTFC) has shown to reduce IOP as compared with their individual components.

In a 3-month, randomized, double-masked study reported by Barnebey et al [181] of TTFC versus its component medications used as monotherapy, 263 patients were treated with TTFC QD in the morning, travoprost QD in the evening, or timolol bid. TTFC reduced IOP substantially more than timolol alone throughout the study. At month 3, the mean reduction from baseline IOP was approximately 1.1 to 2.4 mmHg larger in the TTFC group than in the travoprost group, but the difference was statistically significant at only 2 of 3 time points, and the reductions were measured from a baseline IOP that was approximately 0.6 mmHg higher in the TTFC group. No statistical analysis of adverse events in the study was reported. The incidence of conjunctival hyperemia was 14.1% in the TTFC group, 11.6% in the travoprost group, and 1.1% in the timolol group [181].

Two studies have evaluated the efficacy and safety of TTFC QD in the morning compared with concomitant treatment with travoprost QD in the evening and timolol QD in the morning [182, 183]. In the study reported by Schuman et al [182] the mean reduction from baseline IOP was greater with concomitant therapy than with TTFC by up to approximately 1.0 mmHg at 5 of 9 follow-up time points and statistically similar between groups at the remaining time points. Similarly, in the study reported by Hughes et al27 mean IOPs were significantly lower in the concomitant therapy group than in the TTFC group by up to approximately 1.0 mmHg at 4 of 9 time points during treatment.

Given the similarity of study designs, a pooled analysis was made to further characterize the efficacy of the fixed combination compared to concomitant administration of its components [184].

Differences in mean IOP between groups (fixed combination minus concomitant) ranged from 0.2 to 1.0 mmHg across visits and time points, with upper 95% confidence limits for these differences ranging from 0.7 to 1.5 mmHg thereby satisfying the criterion for non-inferiority (less than or equal to 1.5 mmHg at all 9 time points) [184]. This pooled analysis of two prospective, randomized, controlled clinical trials demonstrates that the fixed combination of travoprost and timolol offers comparable IOP reduction and a similar safety profile to concomitant therapy with travoprost and timolol [184].

Konstas et al evaluated intraocular pressure control over 24 hours using TTFC administered in the morning or evening in primary open-angle and exfoliative glaucoma [185].When treatments were compared directly, evening dosing provided a statistically significant lower 24-hour curve than morning dosing (p = 0.001). Evening dosing also resulted in a lower 24-hour IOP fluctuation than morning dosing (p = 0.0002) and lower peak IOP (p = 0.0003) [185].

Conversely, Denis et al found that the results were similar in the morning group and in the evening group, and their IOP reductions from baseline ranged from 8 to 10 mmHg (32%–38%) and were statistically significant and clinically relevant in both groups [186].

When compared with the DTFC the fixed combination of travoprost/timolol seems to provide a better IOP control. Teus et al compared the intraocular pressure- (IOP-) lowering efficacy of fixed combinations travoprost 0.004%/timolol 0.5% and dorzolamide 2%/timolol 0.5% in patients with ocular hypertension or open-angle glaucoma [187]. This study found that he travoprost/timolol combination produced mean IOP reductions from baseline of 35.3% to 38.5%, while the dorzolamide/timolol combination produced mean IOP reductions from baseline of 32.5% to 34.5%, suggesting a superior mean diurnal IOP-lowering efficacy of TTFC as compared to dorzolamide 2%/timolol 0.5% [187].

3.7.3.3. Fixed Combination of Bimatoprost/Timolol

The prostaglandin analog bimatoprost has been combined with timolol in fixed-combination bimatoprost 0.03%/timolol 0.5% (BiTFC) (Ganfort®; Allergan, Inc.).

Brandt et al [188] of BiTFC versus its component medications used as monotherapy, 1061 patients were treated with BiTFC QD in the morning, bimatoprost QD in the evening, or timolol BID. After 3 months, the mean change from baseline diurnal IOP in the BiTFC group (8.1 mmHg) was larger than in the timolol group (6.4 mmHg) but not the bimatoprost group (7.9 mmHg). Although BiTFC was consistently more effective than timolol at reducing IOP, the mean reduction from baseline IOP was significantly larger with BiTFC than with bimatoprost alone at only 5 of 9 follow-up time points.

Hommer et al in a 3-week, randomized, double-masked, parallel-group study reported that BiTFC QD in the morning reduced IOP as effectively as concomitant treatment with bimatoprost QD in the evening and timolol BID at the 3 follow-up timepoints in the study (hours 1, 2, and 8 at week 3) [189].

BiTFC seems to induce a greater IOP reduction when compared with LTFC [189-191].

Additionally, Centofanti et al in a multicenter, prospective, randomized, double-mask, and cross-over study found that BiTFC provided further IOP reduction in glaucoma patients previously treated with LTFC [193].

Regarding the safety profile, BiTFC seems to have less hyperemia than bimatoprost monotherapy [189].

3.7.4. Adrenergic Antagonist and Topical Carbonic Anhydrase Inhibitors

3.7.4.1. Fixed Combination of Dorzolamide/Timolol

Dorzolamide/timolol (Cosopt®; Merck and Co., Inc.) has been available since 1998 for reducing IOP in patients who do not respond adequately to beta blockers alone, and it has become widely used and accepted.

The IOP-lowering effect of the dorzolamide–timolol fixed combination has been found to be greater than that of either of its components when they are each administered as monotherapy [194, 195].

The efficacy of the dorzolamide–timolol fixed combination (dorzolamide–timolol dosed twice daily) was also found to be comparable to the IOP-lowering effect of its individual components when administered concomitantly (dorzolamide hydrochloride 2% 3 times daily plus timolol maleate 0.5% twice daily).

Hutzelmann et found that DTFC and the no fixed combination of dorzolamide and timolol were equivalent in IOP lowering, with the difference in mean IOP lowering between treatment groups <0.1 mmHg at both peak and trough effect [196].

In contrast, in a 3-month, randomized, double-masked study reported by Strohmaier et al that compared DTFCTID with concomitant dorzolamide TID and timolol TID in 242 patients, DTFC treatment was approximately 1 mmHg less effective than concomitant therapy with dorzolamide and timolol in reducing IOP [197].

Several open-label replacement studies have suggested that patients may achieve additional IOP lowering when they are switched from dorzolamide and a beta-blocker to DTFC [198-201]. It should be noted that Phase IV trials such as these are subject to bias, because the investigators are not masked and the study design may influence the study outcomes.

Numerous clinical studies show comparable efficacy between the fixed combination dorzolamide–timolol and other topical agents used alone or in combination therapies [202].

DTFC is available as a preservative free formulation. The efficacy and tolerability of preservative-free (PF) and preservative-containing (PC) formulations of the dorzolamide/timolol fixed combination in patients with elevated intraocular pressure (IOP) was compared in a parallel, randomized, double-masked, and prospective study [203]. The results of this study suggested that PF and PC DTFC were equivalent in efficacy for change in trough and peak IOP, and had generally similar tolerability [203].

DTFC has shown to have a similar vascular effect to that of dorzolamide.

For instance, Martinez and Sánchez found the fixed combination of dorzolamide/timolol when compared to latanoprost/timolol fixed combination produced statistically similar IOP reductions; however, only the dorzolamide/ timolol combination increased retrobulbar blood flow velocities [178]. This finding was confirmed in two other studies [88, 204, 205].

The safety profile of the fixed combination dorzolamide–timolol is similar to that of its individual components, and no additional tolerability issues have been identified specifically with this fixed combination therapy.

Thus, the role of fixed combination dorzolamide–timolol can be either as a replacement or adjunct therapy when a patient's IOP is not controlled.

3.7.4.2. Fixed Combination of Brinzolamide/Timolol

The brinzolamide/timolol fixed combination (BzTFC](Azarga®, Alcon Laboratories, Inc.) is comprised of the CAI brinzolamide and the beta-blocker timolol and is recommended to be dosed twice daily.

BzTFC has shown to be more effective than its components administered separately.

Kaback et al in a prospective, randomized, double-masked, parallel group, and multicenter study compared the safety and intraocular pressure lowering efficacy of brinzolamide 1%/timolol 0.5% fixed combination with brinzolamide 1% or timolol 0.5% monotherapy in patients with open-angle glaucoma or ocular hypertension [206]. This study found that BzTFC produced statistically significant reductions from baseline ranging from 8.0

to 8.7 mmHg, which were statistically and clinically superior to that of either brinzolamide 1% (5.1-5.6 mmHg) or timolol 0.5% (5.7-6.9 mmHg) [206].

Additionally, BzTFC seems to be as effective as DTFC with fewer side effects.

Manni et al [207] compared the IOP-lowering efficacy of BzTFC and DTFC in patients with open-angle glaucoma or ocular hypertension who required a change in therapy due to elevated IOP while receiving IOP-lowering medication.

The results of this study suggested that the IOP lowering effect of both treatments was significant and equivalent. However, although a similar overall safety profile was observed between the 2 treatment groups, BzTFC showed significantly less ocular irritation than DTFC. In the brinzolamide/timolol group, a higher incidence of blurred vision was reported.

Regarding the safety profile, in a crossover study, Mundorf and colleagues [207] found better comfort scores for BzTFC than for DTFC. Although the follow up in this study was very limited, a majority of patients preferred brinzolamide/timolol.

Until now, the effects of brinzolamide/timolol on ocular blood flow have been unclear. As far as I know, there is not any study that evaluates the effects of the BzTFC on the ocular blood flow.

Martinez et al evaluated the retrobulbar hemodynamic effects of the association of brinzolamide 1% and timolol 0.5% administered twice daily [91].

Based on the results of this study appears that the vascular effect of brinzolamide did not last longer than 6 months in the CRA and 12 months in the SPCA. In addition, brinzolamide did not exert a statistically significant effect upon the blood flow parameters in the OA [91].

3.7.5. Adrenergic Antagonist and Adrenergic Agonist and Topical Carbonic Anhydrase Inhibitors

The fixed combination of timolol/brimonidine/dorzolamide (BDTFC) (Krytantek Ofteno®, Sophia SA de CV, Zapotan, Mexico) has been available in Mexico since 2007.

Up to now, there is only one study that compared the efficacy and safety of BDTFCin ophthalmic solution versus DTFC in patients with open-angle glaucoma or ocular hypertension. The results of this study suggested that the fixed triple combination was significantly more efficient in mean intraocular pressure reduction from baseline throughout the six-month follow-up [208].

4. PRESERVATIVES IN TOPICAL GLAUCOMA DRUG PREPARATIONS

The regulatory agencies recommend that eye drops must contain an antimicrobial agent (preservative) to avoid or to limit microbial proliferation after opening the bottle, which could induce a risk of eye infection as well as changes in the formulation and its action. Preservatives used in ophthalmic preparations belong to a variety of chemical families, including mercury derivatives, alcohols, parabens, EDTA, chlorhexidine, and quaternary ammonium compounds [209]. Effectiveness on microorganisms performed through cytotoxic effects cannot be achieved without a minimal amount of toxicity to tissues where preservatives are applied [210].

The most commonly used preservative in ophthalmic preparations today is benzalkonium chloride (BAK), due to its low allergenic effect and apparently good safety profile. BAK is a nitrogenous cationic surface-acting agent belonging to the quaternary ammonium group. Quaternary ammoniums are bipolar compounds, which are highly hydro soluble and have surfactant properties. They act mainly via their detergent properties, which vary in strength and dissolve the bacterial walls and membranes, and destroy the semipermeable cytoplasmic layer [209].

Ocular surface changes, including burning or stinging sensations, dry eye and tearing, have been described after the long term administration of topical antiglaucoma agents [211]. A prospective epidemiological survey was conducted in 2002 in 4107 glaucoma patients to assess the effects of preserved and preservative-free eye drops on ocular symptoms and conjunctival, corneal and palpebral signs during clinical practice [212]. All symptoms were significantly more prevalent in patients using preserved drops compared with those using preservative-free treatment. The prevalence of signs and symptoms was dose-dependent, increasing with the number of preserved eye drops used. Furthermore, when patients were either switched to preservative-free drugs or given less preservative-containing drugs, all symptoms and signs improved [212]. Similar data were obtained when equivalent studies were performed in Italy, Belgium and Portugal [213]. Although there were some minor differences between the countries, pooled data from a total of 9658 patients also demonstrated that the incidence of ocular signs and symptoms was significantly (p <0.0001) higher in patients receiving preserved eye drops, and that the incidence of these signs and symptoms decreased significantly (p < 0.0001) by switching to a preservative-free formulation or by reducing the amount of preservative-containing treatment [213].Likewise, a total of 20,506 patients from 900 centers across Germany were included in an observational study on dry eye prevalence in glaucoma. Dry eye occurred more frequently in more severe glaucoma cases, when three or more antiglaucoma drugs were used, and increased with the duration of glaucoma disease [214]. Similarly, in the United States, a cross-sectional study evaluated the impact of ocular surface in glaucoma management in patients with open-angle glaucoma or ocular hypertension. Using the Ocular Surface Disease Index for measuring symptoms of dry eye, 59% of patients reported symptoms in at least one eye, qualified as severe in 27% of patients. Schirmer testing showed 61% of patients with decreased tear production in at least one eye. Corneal and conjunctival lissamine green staining showed positive results in 22% of cases. Tear break-up time was decreased in 78% of patients [215].Another observational survey has confirmed the high prevalence of dry eye in glaucoma patients with a clear relationship with the number of eye drops: 39% and 43% of dry eye with two and three drugs, respectively, whereas dry eye was only found in 11% of patients receiving only one eye drop [216]. These last two studies concluded that ocular surface symptoms had a substantial impact on the patients' quality of life, as is well known in dry eye disease irrespective of the cause [217]. The impact on compliance is very likely, although more difficult to assess. In an observational study the high rate of symptoms led to poor patient satisfaction and reduced adherence. Dissatisfied patients also visited their ophthalmologists more frequently [218]. In a survey performed in the US between 2001 and 2004, based on the refilling rate of initial therapy, adverse effects were found the second most common reasons noted by physicians for switching medications after lack of efficacy (19% vs. 43%, respectively) [219].

The development of subconjunctival fibrosis has been reported in patients treated with antiglaucoma medications for a long period of time, most likely resulting from an increase in fibroblast density in the subepithelial substantia propia, related to an increase in inflammatory cells [220-222]. This inflammation of the conjunctiva could consequently induce an increased postoperative fibrosis. Therefore, the use of topical antiglaucoma drugs can be considered as an important risk factor for failure of filtration surgery and whenever possible, improvement of the ocular surface and reduction of inflammation prior to surgery should be considered [223].

The adverse events observed with the use of antiglaucoma medications may result from either an allergic or a toxic reaction. Although allergy can occur in a small proportion of patients, toxicity is probably the predominant cause. The side-effects may be caused by either the active compound of the antiglaucoma medication, or, as is more likely based on the data shown before, the preservatives which are included within the formulation.

Evidence from several animal studies and human cell line experiments supports the hypothesis that antiglaucoma therapies containing the preservative BAK are associated with various adverse reactions on surface and deep ocular tissues.

Tear film is important because it functions as both a lubricating and protective layer. The cornea holds the tear film on its surface, probably with the aid of mucin-producing goblet cells throughout the conjunctiva. Over 30 years ago, it was shown that 0.01% BAK hastened the drying of the precorneal tear film in rabbits. It shortened the length of time taken for dry spots to appear on the corneal surface by a factor of about four [224].

Administration of solutions containing BAK 0.01% has been linked to the infiltration of immunocompetent cells into the limbus and bulbar conjunctiva in rats [225]. The inflammatory reaction was associated with severe damage to the cornea and conjunctiva, including epithelial alterations and keratinization. Several other animal studies have shown that preservatives are linked to the onset of chronic fibrosis in the conjunctiva [226- 228].

It has been studied the effect of different concentrations of BAK (0.1–0.0001%) on a continuous human conjunctival cell line. Benzalkonium chloride at concentrations of 0.1% and 0.05% caused immediate cell lysis. Exposure to 0.01% BAK was associated with cell death within 24 hours, and doses of 0.005–0.0001% induced apoptotic cell death at 24-72 hours in a dose-dependent manner. These findings suggest that BAK at concentrations as low as 0.0001% causes cell death, and that cell destruction is BAK concentration dependent [229].

There are also studies relating BAK exposure to trabecular meshwork cells [230] and crystalin lens epithelial cells damage [231].

Evidence from many clinical studies supports the experimental data from animal studies and human cells, showing also that preservatives can cause detrimental effects on the superficial ocular tissues [221, 224, 232-246]. The conjunctival cytology specimens of patients on long-term antiglaucoma medication also have distinct characteristics, including epithelial keratinization, squamous metaplasia and a reduction in the number of goblet cells [247]. Histomorphological changes to the epithelium can appear as early as 2 weeks after the start of antiglaucoma treatment [248].

The only way to totally eliminate BAK-related side effects, especially in the most sensitive patients, would obviously be to remove BAK from eye drops; however, this raises industrial and regulatory concerns [211].

Single-dose units are the most frequently used preservative-free preparations and depending on the country, some compounds are available: tafluprost, a prostaglandin analog, but mainly beta-blockers, mostly because they came first to generics and could easily be developed. However, some drawbacks have been pointed out regarding single-dose units, such as higher cost and difficult handling, especially in elderly patients. Multidose bottles have therefore been developed, either by allowing preservative filtration through and adsorption on a porous membrane or by using a valve system that hinders penetration of bacteria into the bottle. The ABAK® (Laboratories Théa, France) and COMOD® (Ursapharm, Germany) systems have thus been patented and commercialized with various beta-blockers such as timolol, carteolol, and non antiglaucomatous compounds [249-251].

Extensive research has been conducted to discover and develop less toxic preservatives than BAK and quaternary ammoniums [211].

However, since a preservative must be a potent antimicrobial agent while not being cytotoxic, only very few agents have been proposed and are commercially available. Investigations in rabbit eyes studied the effects of Purite®, a stabilized oxychloro complex, compared with topical BAK-containing antiglaucoma medications [228]. After 30 days, both in the cornea and the conjunctiva, BAK-containing dorzolamide, timolol, and latanoprost produced significantly more changes than did artificial tears containing Purite® and brimonidine Purite® (p <0.001).

Two other approaches have been developed for avoiding BAK as a preservative in a prostaglandin analog solution travoprost, which was preserved with BAK. In U.S.A. travoprost eye drops solution is available with a new preservative system, Sofzia®, composed of boric acid, propylene glycol, sorbitol, and zinc chloride. A toxicological study in conjunctival cells confirmed that Sofzia® preserved travoprost induced significantly less apoptosis and fewer alterations of cell viability and membrane integrity than did BAK-containing latanoprost or travoprost [252]. The third candidate as a preservative that could be a less toxic alternative to BAK is polyquaternium, a polycationic polymer. At least 37 different polymers exist under the polyquaternium designation but polyquaternium-1, Polyquad® is commonly used as a multipurpose solution for contact lens care and showed a good safety and tolerance profile compared to other multipurpose solutions [253]. This compound is currently commercialized in Europe preserving travoprost solution eye drops as an alternative to BAK [254].

5. ADHERENCE: COMPLIANCE AND PERSISTENCE

Patient cooperation with their medication regimen is essential for treating most chronic diseases; glaucoma is no exception. Poor adherence to medication regimens accounts for substantial worsening of disease and increased healthcare costs [255, 256].Diseases such as diabetes, hypertension, and glaucoma are most problematic because they are typically asymptomatic until the late stages. When patients are without symptoms, they may not realize the importance of daily adherence [257]. However, even in very symptomatic diseases requiring radical therapy such as mastectomy, adherence to tamoxifen diminishes to almost 50% at 2 years [258].

Before discussing the impact of adherence with glaucoma management, it is essential to first define adherence, compliance and persistence which are commonly used in the literature to describe behaviors related to medication use and non-pharmacologic interventions. The World Health Organization [259] defines adherence as "the extent to which a person's behavior, taking medication, following a diet and/or executing lifestyle changes, corresponds with agreed recommendations from a healthcare provider."Compliance is similar but defined as the extent to which a person's behavior coincides with the healthcare provider's medical or health advice. Compliance suggests that a person is passively following a health professional's orders versus being actively involved in the treatment process. Because of this, the use of the term compliance has fallen out of favor. WHO notes that adherence requires patients' agreement to the recommendations, making them active partners with health professionals in their own care.

Persistence is defined as the ability of a person to continue taking medications for the intended course of therapy [259]. With chronic diseases, the appropriate course of therapy may be months, years or a person's lifetime. A patient is classified as non-persistent if he or she stops taking a prescription prematurely. Continuing to take any amount of the medication is consistent with the definition of persistence. Non adherence to medication regimens would include not filling a prescription, not refilling a prescription on time, taking an incorrect dose, taking medication at the wrong time or forgetting a dose.

Many studies have evaluated adherence either directly or indirectly [260, 261], but assessing adherence accurately poses a significant challenge [262].

Direct methods of monitoring involve either observing the patient take the medication or measuring concentration of the drug or metabolite in blood or urine. Obviously is not as easy in treating glaucoma. Indirect methods of assessing adherence include physician-estimated patient compliance, patient self-reporting, evaluating pharmacy refill rates (assessed by an index called Medication Possession Ratio, MPR), measuring the amount of medication in the bottle at each visit, utilizing electronic medication monitors, measuring clinical response, or using a patient completed medication diary. Each method has its advantages and disadvantages and no technique is without flaws. Although there is no consensus on the best method for measuring adherence, most of the studies have concluded that physicians are poor at predicting the degree of patient compliance and patients consistently overestimate their degree of adherence [1, 261, 263]. In fact, 95% of patients claimed in one study (Glaucoma Adherence and Persistency Study; GAPS) [261, 264, 265] that they never missed taking drops, despite clear evidence that adherence of these very patients was dramatically lower.

Adherence with glaucoma medications is considerably less than presumed by doctors and many patients fail to attend follow-up appointments, also essential for the successful management of the disease. A systematic literature review, until February 2004, found that the proportions of patients who deviate from their prescribed medication regimen ranged from 5% to 80% [266].

However, there was large incomparability of the studies and no meta-analysis was performed from 34 articles describing 29 studies in the review.

Persistence with glaucoma medication has been found to be low in several studies, varying from 20%[267] to 64% [268].

Several studies have found differences in adherence and persistence by class of ocular hypotensive medication. Prostaglandins have been found to have higher rates of persistence [268-273] than other classes.

The reasons that patients fail to adhere or become non-persistent [274] include cost (especially in an environment without a public health maintenance organization), tolerability, difficulty administering drops (especially in the more aging glaucoma population), denial, lack of education, forgetfulness, schedule (a dose frequency of more than twice daily is associated with greater non-compliance), and travel issues.

Cyclic behavior is common, from "white-coat syndrome", in which patients are best at dosing medication for 5 days prior to an office visit and then decline in compliance over the 30 days following the office visit, [261, 275] to restarting after gaps of several months [276].

Interestingly, no study to date has demonstrated an association between poor compliance and glaucomatous progression [277]. This may in part be due to the fact that glaucoma is a slowly progressive disease; it can take three or more visual fields to accurately document perimetric progression and patient's paper diaries of medication use may not be very accurate in assessing adherence [278]. However, numerous studies have demonstrated that treating ocular hypertension or glaucoma with ocular hypotensive agents delays the onset of primary open-angle glaucoma or progression of visual field loss [5]. Conceptually, based on these prior studies, one can argue that a certain degree of noncompliance with glaucoma treatment should be a risk factor for the progression of visual field loss [279].

Although not curable, glaucoma is a preventable cause of blindness if effective and successful treatment can be provided at the appropriate time [277]. As we have told, patient adherence to the medication is a constant challenge that is now recognized as an essential component of the treatment plan and several studies have demonstrated that patients are more likely to be adherent to their medication if they understand the disease and the rationale for treatment and if their treatment regimen is simplified. The following recommendations are established by the European Glaucoma Society [6] in its guidelines to improve compliance in glaucoma patients:

1. Eye drop instillation should be linked to landmarks of daily routine
2. Teach the patient how to install eye drops correctly: intervals, lid closure, punctual occlusion
3. Written and audiovisual information can be added to verbal education
4. Communicate with the family of the patient
5. Communicate with the family physician

Maximizing patient adherence to medication has the potential to reduce the number of surgical interventions required to treat glaucoma, prevent unnecessary vision loss, and save the overall healthcare system money in the long run.

REFERENCES

[1] Kass MA, Heuer DK, Higginbotham EJ, Johnson CA, Keltner JL, Miller JP et al. The Ocular Hypertension Treatment Study: a randomized trial determines that topical ocular hypotensive medicationdelays or prevents the onset of primary open-angle glaucoma. *Arch. Ophthalmol.* 2002; 120: 701–713.

[2] Gordon MO, Beiser JA, Brandt JD, Heuer DK, Higginbotham EJ, Johnson CA et al. The Ocular Hypertension Treatment Study: baseline factors that predict the onset of primary open-angle glaucoma. *Arch. Ophthalmol.* 2002; 120: 714–720.

[3] Advanced Glaucoma Intervention Study Investigators: The Advanced Glaucoma Intervention Study (AGIS) (7). The relationship between control of intraocular pressure and visual field deterioration. *Am. J. Ophthalmol.* 2000; 130:429–440.

[4]   Lichter PR, Musch DC, Gillespie BW, Guire KE, Janz NK, Wren PA et al(for the CIGTS Study Group). Interim clinical outcomes in the Collaborative Initial Treatment Study comparing initial treatment randomized to medications or surgery. *Ophthalmology* 2001;108(11):1943–1953.

[5]   Heijl A, Leske MC, Bengtsson B, Hyman L, Bengtsson B, Hussein M. Reduction of intraocular pressure and glaucoma progression: results from the Early Manifest Glaucoma Trial. *Arch. Ophthalmol.* 2002; 120: 1268–1279.

[6]   European Glaucoma Society: Terminology and guidelines for Glaucoma. 3.rd ed. (2008), DOGMA, Savona, Italien (www.eugs.org).

[7]   van der Valk R, Webers CAB, Schouten JASG, Zeegers MP, Hendrikse F, Prins MH. Intraocular pressure-lowering effects of all commonly used glaucoma drugs. *Ophthalmology* 2005; 112: 1177-1185

[8]   Realini T, fechtner RD, Atreides RA, Gollance S. The uniocular drug trial and second eye response to glaucoma medications. *Ophthalmology* 2004; 111: 421-6.

[9]   Chaudhary O, Adelman RA, Shields MB. Predicting response to glaucoma therapy in one eye based on response in the fellow eye: the monocular trial. *Arch. Ophthalmol.* 2008; 126: 1216-20.

[10]   Takahashi M, Higashide T, Sakurai M, Sugiyama K. Discrepancy of the intraocular pressure response between fellow eyes in one-eye trials versus bilateral treatment: verification with normal subjects. *J. Glaucoma* 2008; 17: 169-74.

[11]   Realini TD. A prospective, randomized, investigator-masked evaluation of the monocular trial in ocular hypertension or open-angle glaucoma.*Ophthalmology* 2009; 116: 1237-42.

[12]   Bhorade AM. The monocular trial controversy: a critical review: *Curr. Opin. Ophtahlmol.* 2009; 20: 104-9.

[13]   Bhorade AM, Wilson BS, Gordon MO, Palmberg P, Weinreb RN, Miller E et al (from the Ocular Hypertension Treatment Study Group). The utility of the monocular trial. *Ophthalmology* 2010; 117: 2047-2054.

[14]   Realini T, Fechtner RD. 56000 ways to treat glaucoma. *Ophthalmology* 2002; 109:1955-6.

[15]   15.McKee HD, Gupta MS, Ahad MA, Saldaña M, Innes JR. First-choice treatment preferences for primary open-angle glaucoma in the United Kingdom.Eye (Lond). 2005 Aug;19(8):923-4.

[16]   Owen CG, Carey IM, De Wilde S, Whincup PH, Wormald R, Cook DG. The epidemiology of medical treatment for glaucoma and ocular hypertension in the United Kingdom: 1994 to 2003. *Br. J. Ophthalmol.* 2006 Jul;90(7):861-8.

[17]   Tabet R, Stewart WC, Feldman R, Konstas AG. A review of additivity to prostaglandin analogs: fixed and unfixed combinations. *Surv. Ophthalmol.* 2008 Nov;53 Suppl1:S85-92.

[18]   Ritch R, Shileds MB, Krupin T. Chronic open-angle glaucoma: treatment overview. The Glaucomas.2nd ed. St Louis: Mosby-Year Book, Inc, 1996; 1507-1519.

[19]   Fechtner RD, Singh K. Maximal glaucoma therapy. *J. Glaucoma* 2001;10:S73-5.

[20]   Becker B, Petti TH, Gay AJ. Topical epinephrine therapy of open-angle glaucoma. *Arch. Ophthalmol.* 1961; 66: 219.

[21] Jampel HD, Lynch MG, Brown RH, Kuhar MJ, De Souza EB. Beta-adrenergic receptors in human trabecular meshwork.Identification and autoradiographic localization. *Invest. Ophthalmol. Vis. Sci.* 1987 May;28(5):772-9.

[22] Obstbaum SA, Kolker AE, Phelps CD. Low-dose epinephrine: effect on intraocular pressure. *Arch. Ophthalmol.* 1974; 92:118.

[23] Richards JSF, Drance SM. The effect of 2% epinephrine on aqueous dynamics in the human eye. *Can. J. Ophthalmol.* 1967; 2: 259.

[24] Alexander DW, Berson FG, Epstein DL. A clinical trial of timolol and epinephrine in the treatment of primary open-angle glaucoma. *Ophthalmology* 1988; 95:247.

[25] Kohn AN, Moss AP, Hargett NA, Ritch R, Smith H Jr, Podos SM.Clinical comparison of dipivalyl epinephrine and epinephrine in the treatment of glaucoma.*Am. J. Ophthalmol.*. 1979 Feb;87(2):196-201

[26] Kolker AE, Becker B. Epinephrine maculopathy .*Arch Ophathlmol* 1982; 100: 552-562.

[27] Mackool RJ, Muldoon T, Fortier A, Nelson D. Epinephrine-induced cystoid macular edema in aphakic eyes. *Arch. Ophthalmol.*. 1977 May;95(5):791-3.

[28] Thomas JV, Gragoudas ES, Blair NP, Lapus JV. Correlation of epinephrine use and macular edema in aphakic glaucomatous eyes. *Arch. Ophthalmol.* 1978 Apr;96(4): 625-8.

[29] Theodore J, Leibowitz HM. External ocular toxicity of dipivalyl epinephrine.*Am. J. Ophthalmol.*. 1979 Dec;88(6):1013-6.

[30] Coleiro JA, Sigurdsson H, Lockyer JA.Follicular conjunctivitis on Dipivefrin therapy for glaucoma.*Eye* (Lond). 1988;2 (Pt 4):440-2.

[31] Gharagozloo NZ, Relf SJ, Brubaker RF. Aqueous flow is reduced by the alpha-adrenergic agonist, apraclonidine hydrochloride (ALO 2145).*Ophthalmology.* 1988 Sep;95(9):1217-20.

[32] Abrams DA, Robin AL, Pollack IP, deFaller JM, DeSantis L. The safety and efficacy of topical 1% ALO 2145 (p-aminoclonidine hydrochloride) in normal volunteers.*Arch. Ophthalmol.* 1987 Sep;105(9):1205-7.

[33] Robin AL. Short-term effects of unilateral 1% apraclonidine therapy.*Arch. Ophthalmol.* 1988 Jul;106(7):912-5.

[34] Toris CB, Gleason ML, Camras CB, et al. Effects of brimonidine on aqueous humor dynamics in human eyes. *Arch. Ophthalmol.* 1995;113:1514–17.

[35] Quaranta L, Gandolfo F, Turano R, Rovida F, Pizzolante T, Musig A, et al. Effects of topical hypotensive drugs on circadian IOP, blood pressure, and calculated diastolic ocular perfusion pressure in patients with glaucoma. *Invest. Ophthalmol. Vis. Sci.* 2006 Jul;47(7):2917-23.

[36] Liu JH, Medeiros FA, Slight JR, Weinreb RN.Diurnal and nocturnal effects of brimonidine monotherapy on intraocular pressure. *Ophthalmology.* 2010 Nov;117(11):2075-9.

[37] Krupin T, Liebmann JM, Greenfield DS, Ritch R, Gardiner S. (On behalf of the Low-pressure Glaucoma Study Group). A Randomized Trial of Brimonidine Versus Timolol in Preserving Visual Function: Results From the Low-pressure Glaucoma Treatment Study. *Am. J. Ophthalmol.*.2011 Jan 21.[Epub ahead of print].

[38] Schuman JS, Horwitz B Choplin NT, et al. A 1-year study of brimonidine twice daily in glaucoma and ocular hypertension.A controlled, randomized, multicenter clinical trial. *Arch. Ophthalmol.*. 1997;115:847–52.

[39] LeBlanc RP; for the Brimonidine Study Group 2. Twelve-month results of an ongoing randomized trial comparing brimonidine tartrate 0.2% and timolol given twice daily in patients with glaucoma or ocular hypertension. *Ophthalmology*. 1998;105:1960–7.

[40] Katz LJ. Twelve-month evaluation of brimonidine-purite versus brimonidine in patients with glaucoma or ocular hypertension.*J. Glaucoma*. 2002;11:119–26.

[41] Mundorf T, Williams R, Whitcup S, Felix C, Batoosingh A. A 3 month comparison of effi cacy and safety of brimonidine–purite 0.15% and brimonidine 0.2% in patients with glaucoma or ocular hypertension. *J. Ocular. Pharmacol. Ther.* 2003;19:1.

[42] Enyedi LB, Freedman SF. Safety and effi cacy of brimonidine in children with glaucoma. *J. AAPOS*. 2002;5(5):281–4.

[43] Schoene RB, Martin TR, Charan NB, French CL: Timolol induced bronchospasm in asthmatic bronchitis. *JAMA* 245: 1460–1,1981

[44] Diggory P, Heyworth P, Chau G, et al: Improved lung function tests on changing from topical timolol: non-selective beta-blockade impairs lung function tests in elderly patients. *Eye* 1993; 7:661–3.

[45] Shore JH, Fraunfelder FT, Meyer SM: Psychiatric side effects from topical ocular timolol, a beta-adrenergic blocker. *J. Clin. Psychopharmacol.* 1987; 7:264–7.

[46] Bonomi L: Effects of timolol maleate on tear flow in human eyes. *Graefes Arch. Clin. Exp. Ophthalmol.* 1979; 213:19–22.

[47] Nielsen NV, Eriksen JS: Timolol transitory manifestation of dry eyes in long-term treatment. *Acta. Ophthalmol.* (Copenh) 57:418–24, 1979

[48] Stamper RL, Wigginton SA, Higginbotham EJ.Primary drug treatment for glaucoma: beta-blockers versus other medications. *Surv. Ophthalmol.* 2002 Jan-Feb;47(1):63-73.

[49] Phillips CI, Howitt G, Rowlands DJ. Propranolol as ocular hypotensive agent. *Br. J. Ophthalmol.* 1967 Apr;51(4):222-6.

[50] Katz IM, Hubband WA, Getson AJ, et al: Intraocular pressure in normal volunteers following timolol ophthalmic solution. *Invest. Ophthalmol.* 1976; 15:489-492,

[51] Radius RL, Diamond GR, Pollack IP, Langham ME. Timolol.A new drug for management of chronic simple glaucoma. *Arch. Ophthalmol.*. 1978 Jun; 96(6):1003-8.

[52] Coakes RL, Mackie IA, Seal DV: Effects of long-term treatment with timolol on lacrimal gland function. *Br. J. Ophthalmol.* 1981; 65:603-605.

[53] Zimmerman TJ, Kaufman HE.Timolol.A beta-adrenergic blocking agent for the treatment of glaucoma.*Arch. Ophthalmol.*. 1977 Apr;95(4):601-4.

[54] Schenker HW, Yablonski ME, Podos SM, Linder L. Fluorophotometric study of epinephrine and timolol in human subjects. *Arch. Ophthalmol.* 99:1212-1226, 1981.

[55] Zimmerman TJ, Kass MA, Yablonski ME, Becker B. Timolol maleate; efficacy and safety. *Arch. Ophthalmol.* 1979; 97: 656-8.

[56] Boger WP 3rd, Puliafito CA, Steinert RF, Langston DP. Long-term experience with timolol ophthalmic solution in patients with open-angle glaucoma.*Ophthalmology*. 1978 Mar;85(3):259-67.

[57] Soll DB. Evaluation of timolol in chronic open-angle glaucoma.Once a day vs twice a day. *Arch. Ophthalmol.*. 1980 Dec;98(12):2178-81.

[58] Yablonski ME, Novack GD, Burke PJ, Cook DJ, Harmon G. The effect of levobunolol on aqueous humor dynamics.*Exp. Eye Res.* 1987 Jan;44(1):49-54.

[59] Cinotti A, Cinotti D, Grant W, Jacobs I, Galin M, Silverstone D et al. Levobunolol vs timolol for open-angle glaucoma and ocular hypertension. *Am. J. Ophthalmol.*. 1985 Jan 15;99(1):11-7.

[60] The Levobunolol Study Group (Appended). Levobunolol.A beta-adrenoceptor antagonist effective in the long-term treatment of glaucoma. *Ophthalmology* 1985; 92: 1271-76.

[61] Ober M, Scharrer A, David R, Biedner BZ, Novack GD, Lue JC et al. Long-term ocular hypotensive effect of levobunolol: results of a one-year study. *Br. J. Ophthalmol.* 1985 Aug;69(8):593-9.

[62] Wandel T, Charap AD, Lewis RA, Partamian L, Cobb S, Lue JC, et al. Glaucoma treatment with once-daily levobunolol. *Am. J. Ophthalmol.*. 1986 Mar 15;101(3): 298-304.

[63] Rakofsky SI, Lazar M, Almog Y, LeBlanc RP, Mann C, Orr A, et al. Efficacy and safety of once-daily levobunolol for glaucoma therapy. *Can. J. Ophthalmol.*. 1989 Feb;24(1):2-6.

[64] Henness S, Swainston Harrison T, Keating GM.Ocular carteolol: a review of its use in the management of glaucoma and ocular hypertension. *Drugs Aging.* 2007;24(6): 509-28.

[65] Freedman SF, Freedman NJ, Shields MB, Lobaugh B, Samsa GP, Keates EU, et al. Effects of ocular carteolol and timolol on plasma high-density lipoprotein cholesterol level. *Am. J. Ophthalmol.*. 1993 Nov 15;116(5):600-11.

[66] Berrospi AR, Leibowitz HM. Betaxolol. A new beta-adrenergic blocking agent for treatment of glaucoma. *Arch. Ophthalmol.*. 1982 Jun;100(6):943-6.

[67] Reiss GR, Brubaker RF.The mechanism of betaxolol, a new ocular hypotensive agent. *Ophthalmology.* 1983 Nov;90(11):1369-72.

[68] Feghali JG, Kaufman PL.Decreased intraocular pressure in the hypertensive human eye with betaxolol, a beta 1-adrenergic antagonist. *Am. J. Ophthalmol.*. 1985; 15;100(6):777-82.

[69] Caldwell DR, Salisbuty CR, Guzek JP: Effects oftopical betaxolol in ocular hypertensive patients. *Arch. Ophthalmol.* 1984; 102: 539-540.

[70] Radius RL. Use of betaxolol in the reduction of elevated intraocular pressure. *Arch. Ophthalmol.*. 1983 Jun;101(6):898-900.

[71] Allen R. Hertzmark E. walker AM, Epstein DL: A double masked comparison of betaxolol vs. timolol in the treatment of open-angle glaucoma. *Am. J. Ophthalmol.* 1986; 101:535-541.

[72] Allen RC, Epstein DL.Additive effect of betaxolol and epinephrine in primary open angle glaucoma.*Arch. Ophthalmol.*. 1986;104(8):1178-84.

[73] Collignon-Brach J.Long-term effect of ophthalmic beta-adrenoceptor antagonists on intraocular pressure and retinal sensitivity in primary open-angle glaucoma. *Curr. Eye Res.* 1992;11(1):1-3.

[74] Gaul GR, Will NJ, Brubaker RF. Comparison of a noncardioselective beta-adrenoceptor blocker and a cardioselective blocker in reducing aqueous flow in humans. *Arch. Ophthalmol..* 1989;107(9):1308-11.

[75] Ananthanarayan CR, Vaile SJ, Feldman F.Acute episode of asthma following topical administration of betaxolol eyedrops. *Can. J. Ophthalmol..* 1993; 28(2):80-1.

[76] Schoene RB, Abuan T, Ward RL, Beasley CH.Effects of topical betaxolol, timolol, and placebo on pulmonary function in asthmatic bronchitis. *Am. J. Ophthalmol..* 1984 Jan;97(1):86-92.

[77] Van Buskirk EM, Weinreb RN, Berry DP, Lustgarten JS, Podos SM, Drake MM.Betaxolol in patients with glaucoma and asthma. *Am. J. Ophthalmol..* 1986 May 15;101(5):531-4.

[78] Brooks AM, Burden JG, Gillies WE.The significance of reactions to betaxolol reported by patients. *Aust. N. Z. J. Ophthalmol.* 1989; 17(4):353-5.

[79] Innocenti A, Beyza Oztürk Sarikaya S, Gülçin I, Supuran CT. Carbonic anhydrase inhibitors. Inhibition of mammalian isoforms I-XIV with a series of natural product polyphenols and phenolic acids. *Bioorg. Med. Chem.* 2010 Mar 15;18(6):2159-64.

[80] Dobbs PC, Epstein DL, Anderson PJ. Identification of isoenzyme C as the principal carbonic anhydrase in human ciliary processes. *Invest. Ophthalmol. Vis. Sci.* 1979 Aug;18(8):867-70.

[81] Krupin T, Sly WS, Whyte MP, Dodgson SJ. Failure of acetazolamide to decrease intraocular pressure in patients with carbonic anhydrase II deficiency.*Am. J. Ophthalmol..* 1985 Apr 15;99(4):396-9.

[82] Herkel U, Pfeiffer N. Update on topical carbonic anhydrase inhibitors. *Curr Opin Ophthalmol.* 2001 Apr;12(2):88-93.

[83] Pfeiffer N. Dorzolamide: development and clinical application of a topical carbonic anhydrase inhibitor. *Surv. Ophthalmol.* 1997 Sep-Oct;42(2):137-51.

[84] Sugrue MF: The preclinical pharmacology of dorzolamide hydrochloride. a topical carbonic anhydrase inhibitor, *J. Ocul. Pharmacol. Ther.* 1996; 12:363-376.

[85] Lippa EA, Carlson LE, Ehinger B, Eriksson LO, Finnström K, Holmin C, et al. Dose response and duration of action of dorzolamide, a topical carbonic anhydrase inhibitor. *Arch. Ophthalmol.* 1992 Apr;110(4):495-9.

[86] O'Connor DJ, Martone JF, Mead A. Additive intraocular pressure lowering effect of various medications with latanoprost. *Am. J. Ophthalmol..* 2002 Jun;133(6):836-7.

[87] Weinreb RN, Harris, A (Eds.) Ocular Blood Flow in Glaucoma: The 6th Con sensus Report of the World Glaucoma Association. Amsterdam/The Hague, The Netherlands: Kugler Publications 2009, pp. 157-158.

[88] Siesky B, Harris A, Brizendine E, Marques C, Loh J, Mackey J, Overton J, Netland P. Literature review and meta-analysis of topical carbonic anhydrase inhibitors and ocular blood flow. *Surv. Ophthalmol.* 2009 Jan-Feb;54(1):33-46].

[89] Martínez A, Sanchez M. Effects of dorzolamide 2% added to timolol maleate 0.5% on intraocular pressure, retrobulbar blood flow, and the progression of visual field damage in patients with primary open-angle glaucoma: a single-center, 4-year, open-label study. *Clin. Ther.* 2008; 30: 1120-1134.

[90] Martínez A, Sanchez-Salorio M. Predictors for visual field progression and the effects of treatment with dorzolamide 2% or brinzolamide 1% each added to timolol 0.5% in primary open-angle glaucoma. *Acta Ophthalmol.* 2010 Aug;88(5):541-52.

[91] Martínez A, Sánchez-Salorio M. A comparison of the long-term effects of dorzolamide 2% and brinzolamide 1%, each added to timolol 0.5%, on retrobulbar hemodynamics and intraocular pressure in open-angle glaucoma patients. *J. Ocul. Pharmacol. Ther.* 2009 Jun;25(3):239-48.

[92] Pfeiffer N, Grehn F, Hennekes R, Garus H: Augeninnendrucksenkung nach Applikation des lokalen ffirboanhydrasehemmers (MK-297)-Wirkungsvergleich mit Pilocarpin. *Fortschr Ophthalmol* 1990; 87:128-130.

[93] Silver LH. Dose-response evaluation of the ocular hypotensive effect of brinzolamide ophthalmic suspension (Azopt). Brinzolamide Dose-Response Study Group. *Surv. Ophthalmol.* 2000 Jan;44 Suppl 2:S147-53.

[94] March WF, Ochsner KI. The long-term safety and efficacy of brinzolamide 1.0% (azopt) in patients with primary open-angle glaucoma or ocular hypertension.The Brinzolamide Long-Term Therapy Study Group. *Am. J. Ophthalmol..* 2000 Feb;129(2):136-43.

[95] Sall K. The efficacy and safety of brinzolamide 1% ophthalmic suspension (Azopt) as a primary therapy in patients with open-angle glaucoma or ocular hypertension. Brinzolamide Primary Therapy Study Group. *Surv. Ophthalmol.* 2000 Jan;44 Suppl 2:S155-62.

[96] Shin D. Adjunctive therapy with brinzolamide 1% ophthalmic suspension (Azopt) in patients with open-angle glaucoma or ocular hypertension maintained on timolol therapy. *Surv. Ophthalmol.* 2000 Jan;44 Suppl 2:S163-8.

[97] Ishikawa M, Yoshitomi T. Effects of brinzolamide vs timolol as an adjunctive medication to latanoprost on circadian intraocular pressure control in primary open-angle glaucoma Japanese patients. *Clin. Ophthalmol.* 2009;3:493-500.

[98] Kaup M. Plange N. Niegel M., et al. Effects of brinzolamide on ocular haemodynamics in healthy volunteers. *Br. J. Ophthalmol.* 2004;88:257–262.

[99] BECKER B. Diamox and the therapy of glaucoma. *Am. J. Ophthalmol..* 1954 Jul;38(1:1):109-11.

[100] Lehmann B, Linnér E, Wistrand PJ: The pharmacokinetics of acetazolamide in relation to its use in the treatment of glaucoma and its effects as an inhibitor of carbonic anhydrases, In Rospe G, ed: Shering workshop in pharmacokinetics, vol 5, New York, 1970, Pergamon Press.

[101] Linner E, Wistrand P. The initial drop of the intraocular pressure following intravenous administration of acetazolamide in man.Acta Ophthalmol (Copenh). 1959;37:209-14.

[102] Kass MA, Korey M, Gordon M, Becker B. Timolol and acetazolamide. A study of concurrent administration. *Arch. Ophthalmol..* 1982 Jun;100(6):941-2.

[103] Stone RA, Zimmerman TJ, Shin DH, Becker B, Kass MA. Low-dose methazolamide and intraocular pressure. *Am. J. Ophthalmol..* 1977 May;83(5):674-9.

[104] Lichter PR, Newman LP, Wheeler NC, Beall OV. Patient tolerance to carbonic anhydrase inhibitors. *Am. J. Ophthalmol..* 1978 Apr;85(4):495-502.

[105] Lippa EA. Carbonic anhydrase inhibitors. The Glaucomas. 2nd ed. St Louis: Mosby-Year Book, Inc, 1996; 1463-81.

[106] Maren TH. Teratology and carbonic anhydrase inhibition.*Arch. Ophthalmol..*1971 Jan;85(1):1-2.

[107] Nardin GF, Zimmerman TJ. Ocular cholinergic agents.The Glaucomas. 2nd ed. St Louis: Mosby-Year Book, Inc, 1996; 1399-1408.

[108] Weber A. Die ursache des glaukoms, *Graefes Arch. Ophthalmol.* 1877; 23:1.

[109] Drance SM, Nash PA. The dose response of human intraocular pressure to pilocarpine. *Can. J. Ophthalmol.* 1971 Jan;6(1):9-13.

[110] Fry LL. Comparison of the postoperative intraocular pressure with Betagan, Betoptic, Timoptic, Iopidine, Diamox, Pilopine Gel, and Miostat. *J. Cataract Refract Surg.* 1992 Jan;18(1):14-9.

[111] Toris CB, Camras CB, Yablonski ME, et al: Effects of exogenous prostaglandins on aqueous humor dynamics and blood-aqueous barrier function. *Surv. Ophthalmol.* 1997; 41(Suppl 2):S69—75.

[112] Weinreb RN, Toris CB, Gabelt BT, et al: Effects of prostaglandins on the aqueous humor outflow pathways. *Surv. Ophthalmol.* 2002;47(Suppl 1):S53-64.

[113] Alm A, Camras C, Watson P: Phase 3 latanoprost studies in Scandinavia, the United Kingdom, and the United States. *Stow Ophthalmol* 1997; 41 (Suppl 2):S105-S110.

[114] Alm A, Stjernschantz J, Scandinavian Latanoprost StudyGroup: Effects on intraocular pressure and side effects of 0.005% latanoprost once daily, evening or morning. A comparison with timolol. *Ophthahnology* 1995; 102:1743-1752.

[115] Hedman K, Alm A: A pooled data analysis of three randomised, double-masked six-month clinical studies comparing the intraocular pressure reducing effect of latanoprost and timolol. *Eur J Ophthalmol* 2000; 2:94–104.

[116] Hedman K, Alm A, Gross RL. Pooled-data analysis of three randomized, double-masked, six-month studies comparing intraocular pressure-reducing effects of latanoprost and timolol in patients with ocular hypertension. *J. Glaucoma.* 2003 Dec;12(6):463-5.

[117] Alm A, Schoenfelder J, McDermott J. A 5-year, multicenter, open-label, safety study of adjunctive latanoprost therapy for glaucoma. *Arch. Ophthalmol..* 2004 Jul;122(7): 957-65.

[118] Netland PA, Landry T, Sullivan EK, et al. Travoprost compared with latanoprost and timolol in patients with open-angle glaucoma or ocular hypertension. *Am. J. Ophthalmol.* 2001;132:472–484.

[119] DuBiner H, Cooke D, Dirks M, Stewart WC, VanDenburgh AM, Felix C. Efficacy and safety of bimatoprost in patients with elevated intraocular pressure: a 30-day comparison with latanoprost. *Surv. Ophthalmol.* 2001;45(Suppl 4):S353–S360.

[120] Gandolfi S, Simmons ST, Sturm R, Chen K, VanDenburgh AM, for the Bimatoprost Study Group 3. Three-month comparison of bimatoprost and latanoprost in patients with glaucoma and ocular hypertension. *Adv. Ther.* 2001;18:110–121.

[121] Parrish RK, Palmberg P, Sheu WP; XLT Study Group. A comparison of latanoprost, bimatoprost, and travoprost in patients with elevated intraocular pressure: a 12-week, randomized, masked-evaluator multicenter study. *Am. J. Ophthalmol..* 2003 May;135(5):688-703.

[122] Hedman K, Larsson LI. The effect of latanoprost compared with timolol in African-American, Asian, Caucasian, and Mexican open-angle glaucoma or ocular hypertensive patients. *Surv. Ophthalmol.* 2002 Aug;47 Suppl 1:S77-89.

[123] Netland PA, Robertson SM, Sullivan EK, Silver L, Bergamini MV, Krueger S, Weiner AL, Davis AA; Travoprost Study Groups. Response to travoprost in black and nonblack patients with open-angle glaucoma or ocular hypertension. *Adv. Ther.* 2003 May-Jun;20(3):149-63.

[124] Birt CM, Buys YM, Ahmed II, Trope GE; Toronto Area Glaucoma Society. Prostaglandin efficacy and safety study undertaken by race (the PRESSURE study). *J. Glaucoma.* 2010 Sep;19(7):460-7.

[125] Zabriskie N, Netland PA: Comparison of brimonidine/latanoprost and timolol/dorzolamide: two randomized, doublemasked, parallel clinical trials. *Adv. Ther.* 2003; 20:92-100.

[126] Hatanaka M, Vessani RM, Elias IR, Morita C, Susanna R Jr. The effect of prostaglandin analogs and prostamide on central corneal thickness. *J. Ocul. Pharmacol. Ther..* 2009 Feb;25(1):51-3.

[127] Hellberg MR, Sallee VL, McLaughlin MA, et al: Preclinical efficacy of travoprost, a potent and selective FP prostaglandin receptor agonist. *J. Ocul. Pharmacol.* Ther. 2001; 17:421–32.

[128] Hellberg MR, McLaughlin MA, Sharif NA: Identification and characterization of the ocular hypotensive efficacy of travoprost, a potent and selective FP prostaglandin receptoragonist, and AL-6598, a DP prostaglandin receptor agonist. *Surv. Ophthalmol.* 2002; 47(Suppl 1):S13–S33.

[129] Toris CB, Zhan GL, Camras CB, et al: Effects of travoprost on aqueous humor dynamics in monkeys. *J. Glaucoma* 2005; 14: 70-73.

[130] Toris CB, Zhan G, Fan S, et al: Effects of travoprost on aqueous humor dynamics in patients with elevated intraocular pressure. *J. Glaucoma* 2007; 16:189-95.

[131] Goldberg I, Cunha-Vaz J, Jakobsen JE, et al: Comparison of topical travoprost eye drops given once daily and timolol 0.5% given twice daily in patients with open-angle glaucoma or ocular hypertension. *J. Glaucoma* 2001; 10:414–22.

[132] Cantor LB, Hoop J, Morgan L, Wudunn D, Catoira Y; Bimatoprost-Travoprost Study Group. Intraocular pressure-lowering efficacy of bimatoprost 0.03% and travoprost 0.004% in patients with glaucoma or ocular hypertension. *Br. J. Ophthalmol.* 2006 Nov;90(11):1370-3.

[133] Orzalesi N, Rossetti L, Bottoli A, Fogagnolo P. Comparison of the effects of latanoprost, travoprost, and bimatoprost on circadian intraocular pressure in patients with glaucoma or ocular hypertension. *Ophthalmology.* 2006 Feb;113(2):239-46.

[134] Stewart WC, Konstas AG, Nelson LA, Kruft B. Meta-analysis of 24-hour intraocular pressure studies evaluating the efficacy of glaucoma medicines. *Ophthalmology.* 2008 Jul;115(7):1117-1122.e1.

[135] Eisenberg DL, Toris CB, Camras CB. Bimatoprost and travoprost: a review of recent studies of two new glaucoma drugs. *Surv. Ophthalmol.* 2002 Aug;47 Suppl 1:S105-15.

[136] Feldman RM, Tanna AP, Gross RL, Chuang AZ, Baker L, Reynolds A, Prager TC;Additivity Study Group. Comparison of the ocular hypotensive efficacy ofadjunctive brimonidine 0.15% or brinzolamide 1% in combination with travoprost 0.004%. *Ophthalmology.* 2007 Jul;114(7):1248-54.

[137] Franks W: Ocular hypotensive efficacy and safety of brinzolamide ophthalmic suspension 1% added to travoprost ophthalmic solution 0.004% therapy in patients with open-angle glaucoma or ocular hypertension. *Curr. Med. Res. Opin.* 2006; 22:1643-49.

[138] Woodward DF, Krauss AH, Chen J, Lai RK, Spada CS, Burk RM, et al.The pharmacology of bimatoprost (Lumigan). *Surv. Ophthalmol.* 2001 May;45 Suppl 4:S337-45.

[139] Woodward DF, Krauss AH, Wang JW, Protzman CE, Nieves AL, Liang Y, et al. Identification of an antagonist that selectively blocks the activity of prostamides (prostaglandin-ethanolamines) in the feline iris. *Br. J. Pharmacol.* 2007 Feb;150(3):342-52.

[140] Brubaker RF, Schoff EO, Nau CB, Carpenter SP, Chen K, Vandenburgh AM. Effects of AGN 192024, a new ocular hypotensive agent, on aqueous dynamics. *Am. J. Ophthalmol..* 2001 Jan;131(1):19-24.

[141] Brandt JD, VanDenburgh AM, Chen K, Whitcup SM; Bimatoprost Study Group. Comparison of once- or twice-daily bimatoprost with twice-daily timolol in patients with elevated IOP: a 3-month clinical trial. *Ophthalmology.* 2001 Jun;108(6):1023-31.

[142] Faridi UA, Saleh TA, Ewings P, Venkateswaran M, Cadman DH, Samarasinghe RA, Vodden J, Claridge KG. Comparative study of three prostaglandin analogues in the treatment of newly diagnosed cases of ocular hypertension, open-angle and normal tension glaucoma. *Clin. Experiment Ophthalmol.* 2010 Oct;38(7):678-82.

[143] Katz LJ, Cohen JS, Batoosingh AL, Felix C, Shu V, Schiffman RM. Twelve-month, randomized, controlled trial of bimatoprost 0.01%, 0.0125%, and 0.03% in patients with glaucoma or ocular hypertension. *Am. J. Ophthalmol..* 2010 Apr;149(4):661-671.e1.

[144] Brittain CJ, Saxena R, Waldock A, et al: Prospective comparative switch study from timolol 0.5% and latanoprost 0.005% to bimatoprost 0.03%. *Adv. Ther.* 2006; 23:68-73.

[145] Alm A, Grierson I, Shields MB. Side effects associated with prostaglandin analog therapy. *Surv. Ophthalmol.* 2008; 53:S93-S105.

[146] D'Alena P, Ferguson W. Adverse effects after glycerol orally and mannitol parenterally. *Arch. Ophthalmol..* 1966 Feb;75(2):201-3.

[147] Takagi Y, Nakajima T, Shimazaki A, Kageyama M, Matsugi T, Matsumura Y, et al. Pharmacological characteristics of AFP-168 (tafluprost), a new prostanoid FP receptor agonist, as an ocular hypotensive drug. *Exp. Eye Res.* 2004 Apr;78(4):767-76.

[148] Aihara M. Clinical appraisal of tafluprost in the reduction of elevated intraocular pressure (IOP) in open-angle glaucoma and ocular hypertension. *Clin. Ophthalmol.* 2010;4:163–170.

[149] Kanamori A, Naka M, Fukuda M, Nakamura M, Negi A. Tafluprost protects rat retinal ganglion cells from apoptosis in vitro and in vivo. *Graefes Arch. Clin. Exp. Ophthalmol.* 2009 Oct;247(10):1353-60.

[150] Sutton A, Gilvarry A, Ropo A. A comparative, placebo-controlled study of prostanoid fluoroprostaglandin-receptor agonists tafluprost and latanoprost in healthy males. *J. Ocul. Pharm. Ther.* 2007;23:359–365.

[151] Sutton A, Gouws P, Ropo A. Tafluprost, a new potent prostanoid receptor agonist: A dose-response study on pharmacodynamics and tolerability in healthy volunteers. *Int. J. Clin. Pharm. Ther.* 2008;46:400–406.

[152] Uusitalo H, Pillunat LE, Ropo A; Phase III Study Investigators. Efficacy and safety of tafluprost 0.0015% versus latanoprost 0.005% eye drops in open-angle glaucoma and ocular hypertension: 24-month results of a randomized, double-masked phase III study. *Acta Ophthalmol.* 2010 Feb;88(1):12-9.

[153] Kuwayama Y, Komemusi S. Phase III confirmatory study of 0.0015% DE-085 (Tafluprost) ophthalmic solution as compared to 0.005% Latanoprost ophthalmic

solution in patients with open-angle glaucoma or ocular hypertension. *Atarashii Ganka.* 2008;25:1595–1602.

[154] Schnober D, Hofmann G, Maier H, Scherzer ML, Ogundele AB, Jasek MC. Diurnal IOP-lowering efficacy and safety of travoprost 0.004% compared with tafluprost 0.0015% in patients with primary open-angle glaucoma or ocular hypertension. *Clin. Ophthalmol.* 2010 Dec 8;4:1459-63.

[155] Pellinen P, Lokkila J. Corneal penetration into rabbit aqueous humor is comparable between preserved and preservative-free tafluprost. *Ophthalmic. Res.* 2009;41(2):118-22.

[156] Uusitalo H, Kaarniranta K, Ropo A. Pharmacokinetics, efficacy and safety profiles of preserved and preservative-free tafluprost in healthy volunteers. *Acta Ophthalmol.* 2008;86 (Suppl 242):S7–S13.

[157] Hamacher T, Airaksinen J, Saarela V, Liinamaa MJ, Richter U, Ropo A. Efficacy and safety levels of preserved and preservative-free tafluprost are equivalent in patients with glaucoma or ocular hypertension: Results from a pharmacodynamics analysis. *Acta Ophthalmol.* 2008;86(Suppl 242):S14-S19.

[158] Higginbotham EJ. Considerations in glaucoma therapy: fixed combinations versustheir component medications. *Clin. Ophthalmol.* 2010 Feb 2;4:1-9.

[159] Sherwood MB, Craven ER, Chou C, DuBiner HB, Batoosingh AL, Schiffman RM, et al. Twice-daily 0.2% brimonidine-0.5% timolol fixed-combination therapy vs monotherapy with timolol or brimonidine in patients with glaucoma or ocular hypertension: a 12-month randomized trial. *Arch. Ophthalmol.* 2006 Sep;124(9):1230-8.

[160] Goñi FJ; Brimonidine/Timolol Fixed Combination Study Group. 12-week study comparing the fixed combination of brimonidine and timolol with concomitant use of the individual components in patients with glaucoma and ocular hypertension. *Eur. J. Ophthalmol.* 2005 Sep-Oct;15(5):581-90.

[161] Konstas AG, Katsimpris IE, Kaltsos K, Georgiadou I, Kordelou A, Nelson LA, Stewart WC. Twenty-four-hour efficacy of the brimonidine/timolol fixed combination versus therapy with the unfixed components. *Eye* (Lond). 2008 Nov;22(11):1391-7.

[162] Ahmed I. CEED II: an in-depth look at the latest findings. *Clin. Surg. J. Ophthalmol.* 2007;25(1):1–5.

[163] García-Feijoó J, Sáenz-Francés F, Martínez-de-la-Casa JM, Méndez-Hernández C, Fernández-Vidal A, Calvo-González C, et al. Comparison of ocular hypotensive actions of fixed combinations of brimonidine/timolol and dorzolamide/timolol. *Curr. Med. Res. Opin.* 2010 Jul;26(7):1599-606.

[164] Arcieri ES, Arcieri RS, Pereira AC, Andreo EG, Finotti IG, Sá Filho WF. Comparing the fixed combination brimonidine-timolol versus fixed combination dorzolamide-timolol in patients with elevated intraocular pressure. *Curr Med Res Opin.* 2007 Apr;23(4):683-9.

[165] Bill A, Wålinder P-E: The effects of pilocarpine on the dynamics of aqueous humor in a primate (Macaca irus) . *Invest. Ophthalmol* 1966; 5:170-5.

[166] Puustjärvi TJ, Repo LP, The Scandinavian Timpilo Study Group: Timolol-pilocarpine fixed-ratio combinations in the treatment of chronic open angle glaucoma. A controlled multicenter study of 48 weeks. *Arch. Ophthalmol.* 1992; 110:1725-9.

[167] Sturm A, Vogel R, Binkowitz B, The Timolol-Pilocarpine Clinical Study Groups: A fixed combination of timolol and pilocarpine: double-masked comparisons with timolol and with pilocarpine. *J. Glaucoma* 1992; 1:7-13.

[168] Demailly P, Allaire C, Bron V, Trinquand C. Effectiveness and Tolerance of beta-Blocker/Pilocarpine Combination Eye Drops in Primary Open-Angle Glaucoma and High Intraocular Pressure. *J. Glaucoma*. 1995 Aug;4(4):235-41.

[169] Kałuzny JJ, Szaflik J, Czechowicz-Janicka K, Kałuzny J, Orzalkiewicz A,Zaleska A, Krajewska M, Stewart JA, Leech JN, Stewart WC. Timolol0.5%/dorzolamide 2% fixed combination versus timolol 0.5%/pilocarpine 2% fixed combination in primary open-angle glaucoma or ocular hypertensive patients. *Acta Ophthalmol. Scand.* 2003 Aug;81(4):349-54.

[170] Kałuzny J, Sobecki R, Czechowicz-Janicka K, Kecik D, Kałuzny BJ, Stewart JA, et al. Efficacy and safety of latanoprost versus pilocarpine/timolol maleate fixed combination in patients with primary open-angle glaucoma or ocular hypertension. *Acta Ophthalmol.* 2008 Dec;86(8):860-5.

[171] Kass M, Meltzer D, Gordon M, Cooper D, Goldberg J. Compliance with topical pilocarpine treatment. *Am. J. Ophthalmol.* 1986; 101: 515-23.

[172] Higginbotham EJ, Feldman R, Stiles M, Dubiner H; Fixed Combination Investigative Group. Latanoprost and timolol combination therapy vs monotherapy: one-year randomized trial. *Arch. Ophthalmol..* 2002 Jul;120(7):915-22.

[173] Pfeiffer N; European Latanoprost Fixed Combination Study Group. A comparison of the fixed combination of latanoprost and timolol with its individual components. *Graefes Arch. Clin. Exp. Ophthalmol.* 2002 Nov;240(11):893-9.

[174] Higginbotham EJ, Olander KW, Kim EE, Grunden JW, Kwok KK, Tressler CS; United States Fixed-Combination Study Group. Fixed combination of latanoprost and timolol vs individual components for primary open-angle glaucoma or ocular hypertension: a randomized, double-masked study. *Arch. Ophthalmol..* 2010 Feb;128(2):165-72.

[175] Diestelhorst M, Larsson LI; European Latanoprost Fixed Combination Study Group. A 12 week study comparing the fixed combination of latanoprost and timolol with the concomitant use of the individual components in patients with open angle glaucoma and ocular hypertension. *Br. J. Ophthalmol.* 2004 Feb;88(2):199-203.

[176] Diestelhorst M, Larsson LI; European-Canadian Latanoprost Fixed Combination Study Group. A 12-week, randomized, double-masked, multicenter study of the fixed combination of latanoprost and timolol in the evening versus the individual components. *Ophthalmology.* 2006 Jan;113(1):70-6.

[177] Miglior S, Grunden JW, Kwok K; Xalacom/Cosopt European Study Group. Efficacy and safety of fixed combinations of latanoprost/timolol and dorzolamide/timolol in open-angle glaucoma or ocular hypertension. *Eye* (Lond). 2010 Jul;24(7):1234-42.

[178] Martinez A, Sanchez M. Retrobulbar haemodynamic effects of the latanoprost/timolol and the dorzolamide/timolol fixed combinations in newly diagnosed glaucoma patients. *Int. J. Clin. Pract.* 2007 May;61(5):815-25.

[179] Pajic B, Pajic-Eggspuehler B, Häfliger IO. Comparison of the effects of dorzolamide/timolol and latanoprost/timolol fixed combinations upon intraocularpressure and progression of visual field damage in primary open-angle glaucoma. *Curr. Med. Res. Opin.* 2010 Sep;26(9):2213-9.

[180] Rigollet JP, Ondategui JA, Pasto A, Lop L. Randomized trial comparing three fixed combinations of prostaglandins/prostamide with timolol maleate. *Clin. Ophthalmol.* 2011;5:187-91.

[181] Barnebey HS, Orengo-Nania S, Flowers BE, Samples J, Mallick S, Landry TA, et al. The safety and efficacy of travoprost 0.004%/timolol 0.5% fixed combination ophthalmic solution. *Am. J. Ophthalmol.* 2005 Jul;140(1):1-7.

[182] Schuman JS, Katz GJ, Lewis RA, Henry JC, Mallick S, Wells DT, Sullivan EK, Landry TA, Bergamini MV, Robertson SM. Efficacy and safety of a fixed combination of travoprost 0.004%/timolol 0.5% ophthalmic solution once daily for open-angle glaucoma or ocular hypertension. *Am. J. Ophthalmol.* 2005 Aug;140(2):242-50.

[183] Hughes BA, Bacharach J, Craven ER, Kaback MB, Mallick S, Landry TA, et al. A three-month, multicenter, double-masked study of the safety and efficacy of travoprost 0.004%/timolol 0.5% ophthalmic solution compared to travoprost 0.004% ophthalmic solution and timolol 0.5% dosed concomitantly in subjects with open angle glaucoma or ocular hypertension. *J. Glaucoma.* 2005 Oct;14(5):392-9.

[184] Gross RL, Sullivan EK, Wells DT, Mallick S, Landry TA, Bergamini MV. Pooled results of two randomized clinical trials comparing the efficacy and safety of travoprost 0.004%/timolol 0.5% in fixed combination versus concomitant travoprost 0.004% and timolol 0.5%. *Clin. Ophthalmol.* 2007 Sep;1(3):317-22.

[185] Konstas AG, Tsironi S, Vakalis AN, Nasr MB, Stewart JA, Nelson LA, Stewart WC. Intraocular pressure control over 24 hours using travoprost and timolol fixed combination administered in the morning or evening in primary open-angle and exfoliative glaucoma. *Acta Ophthalmol.* 2009 Feb;87(1):71-6.

[186] Denis P, Andrew R, Wells D, Friren B. A comparison of morning and evening instillation of a combination travoprost 0.004%/timolol 0.5% ophthalmic solution. *Eur. J. Ophthalmol.* 2006 May-Jun;16(3):407-15.

[187] Teus MA, Miglior S, Laganovska G, Volksone L, Romanowska-Dixon B, Gos R, et al. Efficacy and safety of travoprost/timolol vs dorzolamide/timolol in patients with open-angle glaucoma or ocular hypertension. *Clin. Ophthalmol.* 2009;3:629-36.

[188] Brandt JD, Cantor LB, Katz LJ, Batoosingh AL, Chou C, Bossowska I; Ganfort Investigators Group II. Bimatoprost/timolol fixed combination: a 3-month double-masked, randomized parallel comparison to its individual components in patients with glaucoma or ocular hypertension. J. Glaucoma. 2008 Apr-May;17(3):211-6. Erratum in: *J. Glaucoma.* 2010 Aug;19(6):423.

[189] Hommer A; Ganfort Investigators Group I. A double-masked, randomized, parallel comparison of a fixed combination of bimatoprost 0.03%/ timolol 0.5% with non-fixed combination use in patients with glaucoma or ocular hypertension. *Eur. J. Ophthalmol.* 2007;17(1):53–62.

[190] Martinez A, Sanchez M. A comparison of the safety and intraocular pressure lowering of bimatoprost/timolol fixed combination versus latanoprost/timolol fixed combination in patients with open-angle glaucoma. *Curr. Med. Res. Opin.* 2007 May;23(5):1025-32.

[191] Martinez A, Sanchez M. Efficacy and safety of bimatoprost/timolol fixed combination in the treatment of glaucoma or ocular hypertension. *Expert Opin. Pharmacother.* 2008 Jan;9(1):137-43.

[192] Martinez A, Sanchez M. Bimatoprost/timolol fixed combination vs latanoprost/timolol fixed combination in open-angle glaucoma patients. *Eye* (Lond). 2009 Apr;23(4):810-8. Epub 2008 Jun 6.

[193] Centofanti M, Oddone F, Gandolfi S, Hommer A, Boehm A, Tanga L, et al. Comparison of Travoprost and Bimatoprost plus timolol fixed combinations in open-angle glaucoma patients previously treated with latanoprost plus timolol fixed combination. *Am. J. Ophthalmol.*. 2010 Oct;150(4):575-80.

[194] Boyle JE, Ghosh K, Gieser DK, Adamsons IA.A randomized trial comparing the dorzolamide-timolol combination given twice daily to monotherapy with timolol and dorzolamide. Dorzolamide-Timolol Study Group. *Ophthalmology.* 1998 Oct;105(10):1945-51.

[195] Clineschmidt CM, Williams RD, Snyder E, Adamsons IA. A randomized trial in patients inadequately controlled with timolol alone comparing the dorzolamide-timolol combination to monotherapy with timolol or dorzolamide. Dorzolamide-Timolol Combination Study Group. *Ophthalmology.* 1998 Oct;105(10):1952-9.

[196] Hutzelmann J, Owens S, Shedden A, Adamsons I, Vargas E; Comparison of the safety and efficacy of the fixed combination of dorzolamide/timolol and the concomitant administration of dorzolamide and timolol: a clinical equivalence study. International Clinical Equivalence Study Group. *Br. J. Ophthalmol.* 1998;82(11):1249–1253.

[197] Strohmaier K, Snyder E, DuBiner H, Adamsons I. The efficacy and safety of the dorzolamide-timolol combination versus the concomitant administration of its components. Dorzolamide-Timolol Study Group. *Ophthalmology.*1998;105(10):1936–1944.

[198] Choudri S, Wand M, Shields MB. A comparison of dorzolamidetimolol combination versus the concomitant drugs. *Am. J. Ophthalmol.*.2000;130(6):832–833.

[199] Martone J, Mead A. Combination treatment may improve efficacy. *Rev Ophthalmol.* 2001;8(September):82–84.

[200] Bacharach J, Delgado MF, Iwach AG. Comparison of the efficacy of the fixed-combination timolol/dorzolamide versus concomitant administration of timolol and dorzolamide. *J. Ocul. Pharmacol. Ther.*.2003;19(2):93–96.

[201] Francis BA, Du LT, Berke S, Ehrenhaus M, Minckler DS; Cosopt Study Group. Comparing the fixed combination dorzolamide-timolol (Cosopt) to concomitant administration of 2% dorzolamide (Trusopt) and 0.5% timolol – a randomized controlled trial and a replacement study. *J. Clin. Pharm. Ther.* 2004;29(4):375–380.

[202] Bell NP, Ramos JL, Feldman RM. Safety, tolerability, and efficacy of fixed combination therapy with dorzolamide hydrochloride 2% and timolol maleate 0.5% in glaucoma and ocular hypertension. *Clin. Ophthalmol.* 2010 Nov 22;4:1331-46.

[203] Shedden A, Adamsons IA, Getson AJ, Laurence JK, Lines CR, et al. Comparison of the efficacy and tolerability of preservative-free and preservative-containing formulations of the dorzolamide/timolol fixed combination (COSOPT™) in patients with elevated intraocular pressure in a randomized clinical trial. *Graefes Arch. Clin. Exp. Ophthalmol.* 2010 Dec;248(12):1757-64.

[204] Siesky B, Harris A, Sines D, Rechtman E, Malinovsky VE, McCranor L, et al. A comparative analysis of the effects of the fixed combination oftimolol and dorzolamide versus latanoprost plus timolol on ocular hemodynamics and visual function in patients with primary open-angle glaucoma. *J. Ocul. Pharmacol. Ther.*. 2006 Oct;22(5):353-61.

[205] Januleviciene I, Harris A, Kagemann L, Siesky B, McCranor L.A comparison of the effects of dorzolamide/timolol fixed combination versus latanoprost on intraocular pressure and pulsatile ocular blood flow in primary open-angle glaucoma patients. *Acta Ophthalmol. Scand.* 2004 Dec;82(6):730-7.

[206] Kaback M, Scoper SV, Arzeno G, James JE, Hua SY, Salem C, Dickerson JE, Landry TA, Bergamini MV; Brinzolamide 1%/Timolol 0.5% Study Group. Intraocular pressure-lowering efficacy of brinzolamide 1%/timolol 0.5% fixed combination compared with brinzolamide 1% and timolol 0.5%. *Ophthalmology.* 2008 Oct;115(10):1728-34, 1734.e1-2.

[207] Mundorf TK, Rauchman SH, Williams RD, Notivol R; Brinzolamide/Timolol Preference Study Group. A patient preference comparison of Azarga (brinzolamide/timolol fixed combination) vs Cosopt (dorzolamide/timolol fixed combination) in patients with open-angle glaucoma or ocular hypertension. *Clin. Ophthalmol.* 2008 Sep;2(3):623-8.

[208] Baiza-Durán LM, Alvarez-Delgado J, Contreras-Rubio AY, Medrano-Palafox J, De Luca-Brown A, Casab-Rueda H, et al. The efficacy and safety of two fixed combinations: timolol-dorzolamide-brimonidine versus timolol-dorzolamide. A prospective, randomized, double-masked, multi-center, 6-month clinical trial. *Ann. Ophthalmol.* (Skokie). 2009 Fall-Winter;41(3-4):174-8.

[209] Vaede D, Baudouin C., Warnet J.-M. and Brignole-Badouin F. Les conservateurs des collyres: vers une prise de conscience de leur toxicité. *J. Fr. Ophtalmol* 2010; 33: 505-524.

[210] Baudouin C. Detrimental effects of preservatives in eyedrops: implications for the treatment of glaucoma. *Acta Ophthalmol.* 2008; 86: 716-726.

[211] Baudouin C., Labbé A, Liang H, Pauly A and Brignole-Baudouin F. Preservatives in eyedrops: The good, the bad and the ugly. *Prog. Retin. Eye Res.* 2010; 29: 312-334.

[212] Pisella P. J., Pouliquen P., Baudouin C. Prevalence of ocular symptoms and signs with preserved and preservative free glaucoma medication. *Br. J. Ophthalmol* 2002; 86: 418-423.

[213] Jaenen N, Baudouin C, Pouliquen P, Manni G, Figueiredo A y Zeyen T. Ocular syntoms and sings with preserved and preservative-free glaucoma medications. *Eur J Ophthalmol* 2007; 17: 341-349.

[214] Erb C, Gast U., Schremmer D. German register for glaucoma patients with dry eye. I. Basic outcome with respect to dry eye. *Graefes Arch. Clin. Exp. Ophthalmol.* 2008; 246: 1593-1601.

[215] Leung EW, Medeiros FA, Weinreb RN. Prevalence of ocular surface disease in glaucoma patients. *J. Glaucoma* 2008: 17: 350-355.

[216] Rossi G.C., Tinelli C., Pasinetti G.M., Milano G., Bianchi P.E. Dry eye syndrome-related quality of life in glaucoma patients. *Eur. J. Ophthalmol.* 2009; 19: 572-579.

[217] Dry Eye Work Shop. The epidemiology of dry eye disease: report of the Epidemiology Subcommittee of the International Dry Eye Work Shop (2007). *Ocul. Surf.* 2007; 5: 93-107.

[218] Nordmann JP, Auzanneau N, Ricard S y Berdeaux G. Vision-related quality of life and topical glaucoma treatment side-effects. *Health Qual. Life Outcomes* 2003; 1: 75.

[219] Zimmermann TJ, Hahn SR, Gelb L, Tan HK, Kim EE and Shah SN. The impact of ocular adverse effects in patients treated with topical prostaglandin analogs: changes in prescription patterns and patient persistence. *J. Ocul. Pharmacol. Ther.* 2009: 25: 145-152.

[220] Baudouin C., Pisella P.J., Fillacier K., Goldschild M., Becquet F., De Saint Jean M., Bechetoille A. Ocular surface inflammatory changes induced by topical antiglaucoma drugs: human and animal studies. *Ophthalmology* 1999; 106: 556-563.

[221] Broadway DC, Grierson I, O'Brien C, Hitchings RA. Adverse effects of topical antiglaucoma medication: the conjuntival cell profile. *Arch. Ophthalmol.* 1994; 112: 1437-45.

[222] Sherwood M.B., Grierson I., Millar L., Hitchings R.A. Long-term morphologic effects of antiglaucoma drugs on the conjunctiva and Tenon's capsule in glau- comatous patients. *Ophthalmology* 1989; 96: 327-335.

[223] Broadway DC y Chang LP. Trabeculectomy, risk factors for failure and the preoperative state of the conjuntiva. *J. Glaucoma* 2001; 10; 237-249.

[224] Wilson W.S., Duncan A.J., Jay J.L. Effect of benzalkonium chloride on the stability of the precorneal tear film in rabbit and man. *Br. J. Ophthalmol.* 1975; 59: 667-669.

[225] Becquet F, Goldschild M, Moldovan MS, Ettaiche M, Gastaud P and Baudouin C. Histopathological effects of topical ophthalmic preservatives on rat corneoconjunctival surface. *Curr. Eye Res.* 1998; 17: 419–425.

[226] Mietz H, Niesen U and Krieglstein GK. The effect of preservatives and antiglaucomatous medication on the histopathology of the conjunctiva.*Graefes Arch. Clin. Exp. Ophthalmol.* 1994; 232: 561–565.

[227] Mietz H, Schlotzer-Schrehardt U, Lemke JH and Krieglstein GK. Early conjunctival changes following treatment with metipranolol and preservatives are not reversible with dexamethasone. *Graefes Arch. Clin. Exp. Ophthalmol.* 1997 235: 452–459.

[228] Noecker RJ, Herrygers LA and Anwaruddin R.: Corneal and conjunctival changes caused by commonly used glaucoma medications. *Cornea* 2004; 23: 490–496.

[229] De Saint Jean M., Brignole F.,Bringuier A.F., Bauchet A., Feldmann G., Baudouin C. Effects of benzalkonium chloride on growth and survival of Chang conjunctival cells. *Invest. Ophthalmol. Vis. Sci.* 1999; 40: 619-630.

[230] Hamard P., Blondin C., Debbasch C., Warnet J.M., Baudouin C., Brignole F. In vitro effects of preserved and unpreserved antiglaucoma drugs on apoptotic marker expression by human trabecular cells. *Graefes Arch. Clin. Exp. Ophthalmol.* 2003; 241: 1037-1043.

[231] Goto Y, Ibaraki N y Miyake K. Human lens epithelial sell damage and stimulation of their secretion of chemical mediators by benzalkonium chloride rather than latanoprost and timolol. *Arch. Ophthalmol.* 2003; 121: 835-839.

[232] Herreras J.M., Pastor J.C., Calonge M., Asensio V.M. Ocular surface alteration after long-term treatment with an antiglaucomatous drug. *Ophthalmology* 1992; 99: 1082-1088.

[233] Baudouin C., Garcher C., Haouat N., Bron A., Gastaud P. Expression of inflammatory membrane markers by conjunctival cell sinchronically treated patients with glaucoma. *Ophthalmology* 1994; 101: 454-460.

[234] de Jong C., Stolwijk T., Kuppens E., de Keizer R., van Best J. Topical timolol with and without benzalkonium chloride: epithelial permeability and autofluorescence of the cornea in glaucoma. *Graefes Arch. Clin. Exp. Ophthalmol.* 1994; 232: 221-224.

[235] Kuppens E.V., de Jong C.A., Stolwijk T.R., de Keizer R.J., van Best J.A. Effect of timolol with and without preservative on the basal tear turnover in glaucoma. *Br. J. Ophthalmol.* 1995; 79: 339-342.

[236] Yalvac I.S., Gedikoglu G., Karagoz Y., Akgun U., Nurozler A., Koc F., Kasim R., Duman S. Effects of antiglaucoma drugs on ocular surface. *Acta Ophthalmol. Scand.* 1995; 73: 246-248.

[237] Baudouin C., de Lunardo C. Short-term comparative study of topical 2% carteolol with and without benzalkonium chloride in healthy volunteers. *Br. J. Ophthalmol.* 1998; 82: 39-42.

[238] Nuzzi R., Finazzo C., Cerruti A. Adverse effects of topical antiglaucomatous medications on the conjunctiva and the lachrymal (Brit.Engl) response. *Int. Ophthalmol.* 1998; 22: 31-35.

[239] Levrat F, Pisella PJ and Baudouin C. Clinical tolerance of antiglaucoma eyedrops with and without a preservative. Results of an unpublished survey in Europe. *J. Fr. Ophtalmol.* 1999; 22: 186–191.

[240] Albietz JM and Bruce AS. The conjunctival epithelium in dry eye subtypes: effect of preserved and non-preserved topical treatments. *Curr. Eye Res.* 2001; 22: 8–18.

[241] Eleftheriadis H, Cheong M, Sandeman S, Syam PP, Brittain P, Klintworth GK, Lloyd A and Liu C. Corneal toxicity secondary to inadvertent use of benzalkonium chloride preserved viscoelastic material in cataract surgery. *Br. J. Ophthalmol.* 2002; 86: 299–305.

[242] Dogan AL, Orhan M, So¨ ylemezoglu F, Irkec, M and Bozkurt B. Effects of topical antiglaucoma drugs on apoptosis rates of conjunctival epithelial cells in glaucoma patients. *Clin. Experiment. Ophthalmol.* 2004; 32: 62–66.

[243] Pisella PJ, Debbasch C, Hamard P, Creuzot- Garcher C, Rat P, Brignole F and Baudouin C. Conjunctival proinflammatory and proapoptotic effects of latanoprost and preserved and unpreserved timolol: an ex vivo and in vitro study. *Invest. Ophthalmol. Vis. Sci.* 2004; 45: 1360–1368.

[244] Kozobolis VP, Detorakis ET, Maskaleris G, Koukoula SC, Fountoulakis N, Chrysochoou F and Konstas AG. Corneal sensitivity changes following the instillation of latanoprost, bimatoprost, and travoprost eyedrops. *Am. J. Ophthalmol.* 2005; 139: 742–743.

[245] Manni G, Centofanti M, Oddone F, Parravano M and Bucci MG. Interleukin- 1beta tear concentration in glaucomatous and ocular hypertensive patients treated with preservative-free non-selective betablockers. *Am. J. Ophthalmol.* 2005; 139: 72–77.

[246] Hong S, Lee CS, Seo KY, Seong GJ and Hong YJ. Effects of topical antiglaucoma application on conjunctival impression cytology specimens. *Am. J. Ophthalmol.* 2006; 142: 185–186.

[247] Costagliola C, Prete AD, Incorvaia C, Fusco R, Parmeggiani F and Di Giovanni A. Ocular surface changes induced by topical application of latanoprost and timolol: a short-term study in glaucomatous patients with and without allergic conjunctivitis. *Graefes Arch. Clin. Exp. Ophthalmol.* 2001; 239: 809–814.

[248] Lewis RA, Katz GJ, Weiss MJ et al. Travoprost 0.004% with and without benzalkonium chloride: a comparison of safety and efficacy. *J. Glaucoma* 2007; 16: 98–103.

[249] Meloni, M., Pauly, A., Servi, B.D., Varlet, B.L., Baudouin, C. Occludin gene expression as an early in vitro sign for mild eye irritation assessment. Toxicol In Vitro 2010; 24: 276-85.

[250] Pisella P.J., Fillacier K., Elena P.P., Debbasch C., Baudouin C. Comparison of the effects of preserved and unpreserved formulations of timolol on the ocular surface of albino rabbits. *Ophthalmic. Res.* 2000; 32: 3-8.

[251] Teping C., Wiedemann B. The COMOD system.A preservative-free multidose container for eyedrops.*Klin. Monbl. Augenheilkd.* 1994; 205: 210-217.

[252] Baudouin C., Riancho L., Warnet J.M., Brignole F. In vitro studies of anti-glaucomatous prostaglandin analogues: travoprost with and without benzal- konium chloride and preserved latanoprost. *Invest. Ophthalmol. Vis. Sci.* 2007; 48: 4123-4128.

[253] Lipener C. A randomized clinical comparison of OPTI-FREE EXPRESS and ReNu MultiPLUS multipurpose lens care solutions. *Adv. Ther.* 2009; 26: 435-446.

[254] Brignole-Baudouin F, Riancho L, Liang H, Nakib Z, Baudouin C. In Vitro Comparative Toxicology of Polyquad-Preserved and Benzalkonium Chloride-Preserved Travoprost/Timolol Fixed Combination and Latanoprost/Timolol Fixed Combination.J. *Ocul. Pharmacol. Ther.*. 2011 Mar 16. [Epub ahead of print].

[255] Rodgers PT, Ruffin DM. Medication non adherence: Part II - a pilot study in patients with congestive heart failure. *Manag Care Interface* 1998; 11: 67-9, 75.

[256] Schiff GD, Fung S, Speroff T, McNutt RA. "Decompensated heart failure: Symptoms, patterns of onset, and contributing factors. *Am. J. Med.* 2003; 114: 625-30.

[257] Schwartz GF. Compliance and persistency in glaucoma follow-up treatment. *Curr. Opin. Ophthalmol.* 2005; 16: 114-21.

[258] Barron TI, Connolly RM, Bennett K, Feely J, Kennedy MJ. Early Discontinuation of Tamoxifen: A Lesson for Oncologists. *Cancer* 2007;109:832-9.

[259] Sabate E. Adherence to Long-Term Therapies: Evidence for Action. Geneva: World Health Organization, 2003. Available from: http://www.who.int/chronic_conditions/ en/adherence_report.pdf.

[260] Okeke CO, Quigley HA, Jampel HD, Ying GS, Plyler RJ, Jiang Y, et al. Adherence with Topical Glaucoma Medication Monitored Electronically: The Travatan Dosing Aid Study. *Ophthalmology* 2009;116:191-9.

[261] Friedman DS, Quigley HA, Gelb L, Tan J, Margolis J, Shah SN, et al. Using Pharmacy Claims Data to Study Adherence to Glaucoma Medications: Methodology and Findings of the Glaucoma Adherence and Persistency Study (GAPS). *Invest. Ophthalmol. Vis. Sci.* 2007; 48: 5052-7.

[262] Schwartz GF and Quigley HA.Adherence and Persistence with Glaucoma Therapy. *Sur. Ophthalmol.* 2008; 53: S57-S68.

[263] Osterberg L, Blaschke T. Adherence to Medication. N Engl J Med 2005; 353: 487-97.

[264] Friedman DS, Hahn SR, Gelb L, et al; Doctor-patient communication and health-related beliefs: Results from the Glaucoma Adherence and Persistency Study (GAPS). *Ophthalmology* 2008; 115:1320-7.

[265] Quigley HA, Friedman DS, Hahn SR: Evaluation of practice patterns for the care of open-angle glaucoma compared with claims data: the Glaucoma Adherence and Persistency Study. *Ophthalmology* 2007; 114:1599-606.

[266] Olthoff CM, Schouten JS, van de Borne BW, Webers CA. Noncompliance with ocular hypotensive treatment in patients with glaucoma or ocular hypertension an evidence-based review. *Ophthalmology.* 2005 Jun;112(6):953-61.

[267] Spooner JJ, Bullano MF, Ikeda LI, et al: Rates of discontinuation and change of glaucoma therapy in a managed care setting. *Am. J. Manag. Care* 2002; 8: S262—70.

[268] Dasgupta S, Oates V, Bookhart BK, et al: Population-based persistency rates for topical glaucoma medications measured with pharmacy claims data. *Am. J. Manag. Care* 2002; 8: S255-61.

[269] Diestelhorst M, Schaefer CP, Beusterien KM, et al: Persistency and clinical outcomes associated with latanoprost and beta-blocker monotherapy: evidence from a European retrospective cohort study. *Eur. J. Ophthalmol.* 2003; 13(Suppl 4): S21—9.

[270] Nordstrom BL, Friedman DS, Mozaffari E, et al: Persistence and adherence with topical glaucoma therapy. *Am. J. Ophthalmol.* 2005; 140:598—606.

[271] Reardon G, Schwartz GF, Mozaffari E: Patient persistency with ocular prostaglandin therapy: a population-based, retrospective study. *Clin. Ther.* 2003; 25:1172—85.

[272] Reardon G, Schwartz GF, Mozaffari E: Patient persistency with topical ocular hypotensive therapy in a managed care population. *Am. J. Ophthalmol.* 2004; 137:S3—12.

[273] Schwartz GF, Reardon G, Mozaffari E: Persistency with latanoprost or timolol in primary open-angle glaucoma suspects. *Am. J. Ophthalmol.* 2004; 137:S13—6.

[274] Tsai JC. A comprehensive perspective on patient adherence to topical glaucoma therapy.*Ophthalmology* 2009; 116: S30-S36.

[275] Feinstein AR: On white-coat effects and the electronic monitoring of compliance. *Arch. Intern. Med.* 1990; 150:1377—8.

[276] Schwartz GF, Platt R, Reardon G, et al: Accounting for restart rates in evaluating persistence with ocular hypotensives. *Ophthalmology* 2007; 114: 648—52.

[277] Robin A and Grover DS. Compliance and adherence in glaucoma management. *Indian J. Ophthalmol.* 2011; 59: 93-96.

[278] Stone AA, Shiffman S, Schwartz AE, Broderick JE, Hufford MR. Patient Non-Compliance with Paper Diaries. *Brit. Med. J.* 2002; 324: 1193-4.

[279] Robin AL, Covert D. Does Adjunctive Glaucoma Therapy Affect Adherence to the Initial Primary Therapy? *Ophthalmology* 2005; 112: 863-8.

In: Glaucoma: Etiology, Pathogenesis and Treatments
Editors: Z. G. Fei and S. Zeng

ISBN: 978-1-61470-975-6
© 2012 Nova Science Publishers, Inc.

Chapter II

Melatonin Protects the Retina from Glaucomatous Damage

Ruth E. Rosenstein*, María C. Moreno, Pablo Sande,
Nuria de Zavalía, Mónica Chianelli, María Inés Keller Sarmiento and
Nicolás Belforte

Laboratory of Retinal Neurochemistry and Experimental Ophthalmology,
Department of Human Biochemistry, School of Medicine,
University of Buenos Aires/CEFyBO, CONICET,
Buenos Aires, Argentina

ABBREVIATIONS

AA-NAT: arylalkylamine N-acetyltransferase;
BDNF: brain-derived neurotrophic factor;
CAT: cationic amino acid transporter;
EAAT-1: excitatory amino acid transporter type 1;
GAD: glutamic acid decarboxylase;
GATs: GABA transporters;
GPX: glutathione peroxidase;
GS: glutamine synthetase;
HA: hyaluronic acid;
HIOMT: hydroxyindole-O-methyltransferase;
iNOS; inducible NOS or NOS-2;
IOP: intraocular pressure;
MT1: melatonin receptor type 1;
MT2: melatonin receptor type 2;

* Corresponding author: Dr. Ruth E. Rosenstein, Departamento de Bioquímica Humana, Facultad de Medicina, CEFyBO Paraguay 2155, 5°P, (1121), Universidad de Buenos Aires, CONICET Buenos Aires, ARGENTINA, phone n°: 54-11-4508-3672 (ext. 37), FAX n°: 54-11-4508-3672 (ex). e-mail: ruthr@fmed.uba.ar

MT3: melatonin receptor type 3;
NMDA: N-methyl D-aspartate;
NOS: NO synthase;
nNOS: neuronal NOS or NOS-1;
ONH: optic nerve head;
POAG: primary open-angle glaucoma;
QR2: quinone reductase 2;
RGC: retinal ganglion cell;
ROS: reactive oxygen species;
SCN: suprachiasmatic nuclei;
SOD: superoxide dismutase.

ABSTRACT

Glaucoma is a complex disease with a number of risk factors and mechanisms which lead to retinal ganglion cell (RGC) death. Ocular hypertension is probably the most important risk factor for primary angle open glaucoma, the more frequent form of glaucoma. However, other factors such as excitotoxicity, reduced antioxidant defense system activity, and an increase in the nitridergic pathway activity have been suggested as possible additional causes for glaucomatous damage. The current management of glaucoma is mainly directed at the control of intraocular pressure (IOP); however, a therapy that prevents the death of RGCs and optic nerve head fiber loss should be the main goal of treatment. In recent years, melatonin has been identified as a neuroprotector in experimental animal models of various neurological and neurodegenerative disorders. In this chapter, we will consider evidence supporting that melatonin, a very safe compound for human use, should be regarded as a new therapeutic resource for the management of glaucoma.

1. BACKGROUND

Melatonin is a ubiquitous natural substance widely distributed in nature, being found both in plants and animals (Pandi-Perumal et al., 2006; Reiter et al., 2007). Melatonin is probably one of the first biologically significant compounds that appeared in living organisms. Although in all mammals, including humans, melatonin is primarily synthesized in the pineal gland, its synthesis also occurs in other tissues, such as bone marrow, gut, gastrointestinal tract, lymphocytes, and in various parts of the eye, i.e. the retina (Cardinali and Rosner, 1971a, 1971b; Faillace et al., 1995; Tosini and Menaker, 1998), the ciliary body (Martin et al., 1992) and the lachrymal gland (Mhatre et al., 1988). In the eye, melatonin which can be locally synthesized or entering from the circulation may contribute to the regulation of retinomotor movements (Pierce and Besharse, 1985), rod outer segment disc shedding (White and Fisher, 1989), dopamine release (Dubocovich, 1983), and intraocular pressure (IOP) (Samples et al., 1988), among many other effects. Moreover, melatonin is an effective antioxidant and free radical scavenger (Siu et al., 2006; Lundmark et al., 2006; Lundmark et al., 2007; Alarma-Estrany and Pintor, 2007, Belforte et al., 2010) which protects the photoreceptor outer segment from oxidative damage induced by light (Siu et al., 1999; Marchiafava and Longoni, 1999).

Glaucoma is a leading cause of blindness worldwide, characterized by specific visual field defects due to the loss retinal ganglion cells (RGCs) and damage to the optic nerve head (ONH). It is estimated that half of those affected may be not aware of their condition because symptoms may not occur during the early stages of the disease. When vision loss appears, considerable and permanent damage has already occurred. Medications and surgery can help to slow the progression of some forms of the disease, but at present, there is no cure. Although an increase in IOP definitely plays a causal role in glaucomatous neuropathy, other factors such as a glutamate excitotoxicity (Moreno et al, 2005a), decrease in GABA levels (Moreno et al., 2008), reduced antioxidant defense system activity (reviewed by Aslan et al., 2008, and Tezel, 2006), and an increase in the nitridergic pathway activity (Neufeld et al., 1999; Belforte et al., 2007) have been suggested as possible additional causes for early stage of glaucomatous damage. The current management of glaucoma is mainly directed at the control of IOP; however, a therapy that prevents the death of ganglion cells should be the main goal of treatment.

Unraveling which are the most critical mechanisms involved in glaucoma is unlikely to be achieved in studies which are limited to the clinically observable changes to the retina and optic nerve head (ONH) that are seen in human glaucoma. Far more detailed and invasive studies are required, preferably in a readily available animal model. An experimental model system of pressure-induced optic nerve damage would greatly facilitate the understanding of the cellular events leading to RGC death, and how they are influenced by IOP and other risk factors associated to glaucoma. Several groups have developed various ways to increase IOP in the rat eye, generally by impeding the outflow of aqueous humor (Shareef et al., 1995; Morrison et al., 1997; Ueda et al., 1998). All of these models have both advantages and disadvantages. We have developed a new model of glaucoma in rats through the intracameral injection of 1% hyaluronic acid (HA). Weekly injections of HA in the rat anterior chamber significantly increase IOP as compared with vehicle-injected contralateral eye (Benozzi et al., 2002; Moreno et al., 2005b). Although multiple injections of HA may be needed to obtain a sustained hypertension, we have shown that the injection procedure itself does not affect IOP and retinal function and histology. On the contrary, several advantages support our model: 1) a highly consistent hypertension is achieved, 2) it may have a reasonably long course, 3) daily variations in IOP persist in HA-injected eyes, 4) in contrast to other models, in all likelihood, HA does not impede the blood flow out of the eye, and 5) it is easy to perform. Furthermore, we have shown that this model may also be utilized for pharmacological studies since the HA-induced hypertension was significantly reduced by the topic and acute application of hypotensive drugs (Benozzi et al., 2002). We have demonstrated that the chronic administration of HA significantly decreases the scotopic electroretinographic activity and provokes a significant loss of RGCs and optic nerve fibers (Moreno et al., 2005b). Based on both functional and histological evidences, these results indicate that the intracameral injections of HA appear to mimic some key features of primary open-angle glaucoma (POAG), and therefore it may be a useful tool to understand this ocular disease and to develop new therapeutic strategies.

Despite the fact that glaucoma is a highly prevalent and major cause of blindness, there are currently no optimal treatments for this ocular disease. In recent years, melatonin has been identified as a neuroprotector in experimental animal models of various neurological and neurodegenerative disorders (Reiter et al., 1999; Srinivasan et al., 2005, 2006). In this context, we will consider evidence supporting that melatonin should be regarded as an important ophthalmic therapeutic resource, particularly for the management of glaucoma.

2. MELATONIN BIOSYNTHESIS IN THE EYE

In most mammals, melatonin is synthesized intraocularly through the same pathway which occurs in the pineal gland (Axelrod, 1974). Tryptophan taken up from the blood is converted into serotonin, which is subsequently metabolized to N-acetyl serotonin by the enzyme arylalkylamine N-acetyltransferase (AA-NAT). N-acetyl serotonin is then converted into melatonin by the enzyme hydroxyindole-O-methyltransferase (HIOMT).

The earliest finding supporting melatonin's biosynthetic pathway in the mammalian retina was the description of HIOMT activity (Cardinali and Rosner, 1971a), and the demonstration that labeled serotonin is converted into melatonin in the rat retina (Cardinali and Rosner, 1971b). The presence of HIOMT in the chicken retina at both protein and mRNA level has been confirmed (Bernard et al., 1999; Liu et al., 2004). The gene encoding HIOMT is selectively expressed in retinal photoreceptors. AA-NAT levels show a circadian rhythm, peaking at night in the chicken and rat retina (Niki et al., 1998; Iuvone et al., 2002). The presence of AA-NAT in the human eye has been well documented (Coon et al., 1996). In the rhesus monkey, AA-NAT activity in pineal and retina shows more than a four-fold increase at night (Coon et al., 2002).

Melatonin biosynthesis in the golden hamster retina is regulated by the light/dark cycle (Faillace et al., 1995). In addition, the finding that isolated *Xenopus* photoreceptor cells rhythmically secrete melatonin suggests that photoreceptors contain an endogenous circadian clock which regulates melatonin biosynthesis (Cahill and Besharse, 1993). This hypothesis has been confirmed in the golden hamster and mouse retinas (Tosini and Menaker, 1996, 1998). In fact, several genes identified as components of the core oscillator in the suprachiasmatic nuclei (SCN) have also been localized in the retina. The clock genes Cryptochrome 1 and 2 are expressed in chicken inner retinal neurons and in the ganglion cell layer (Haque et al., 2002; Bailey et al., 2002). Furthermore, clock genes Period 1 and Period 2 have been identified in the rat retina inner nuclear layer (Namihira et al., 2001), and in a few RGCs of the mouse and human retina (Witkovsky et al., 2003; Thompson et al., 2004). At present, it is not known whether the circadian rhythms in mammalian photoreceptors are driven by inner retinal clocks (Guido et al., 2010). Experiments with the rodless mouse have shown that melatonin synthesis is not abolished by the complete loss of photoreceptors, but that its circadian expression disappears (Tosini, 2000; Tosini and Menaker, 1998). This finding suggests that rods are necessary for the rhythmic synthesis of melatonin. However, more recent evidence indicates that chick RGCs are able to rhythmically synthesize melatonin, even in isolated conditions (Garbarino-Pico et al., 2004).

Regulated by the interaction between a circadian clock and the photic information, retinal melatonin levels rise rapidly after the onset of darkness and decrease after light exposure in the golden hamster and rat (Faillace et al., 1994; Fukuhara et al., 2001). The entire sequence of events has been elegantly studied in chicken photoreceptor cells. The depolarization of photoreceptors that occurs during darkness induces AA-NAT activity by a Ca^{2+} and cAMP dependent mechanism (Ivanova and Iuvone, 2003). Depolarization of the photoreceptor membrane opens dihydropyridine sensitive voltage-gated Ca^{2+} channels resulting in sustained increases in intracellular Ca^{2+} concentrations in the inner segments of photoreceptors, which in turn stimulate cAMP formation through activation of a calmodulin-dependent adenyl cyclase (Gan et al., 1995). Increased levels of cAMP induce AA-NAT gene transcription and increase its activity causing an augmented production of melatonin (Alonso-Gómez and Iuvone, 1995; Greve et al., 1999). Stability of AA-NAT is regulated by cAMP and light, and decreasing cAMP levels in photoreceptor cells, results in rapid degradation of AA-NAT protein by proteasomal proteolysis (Tosini et al., 2006). As for the regulation of melatonin biosynthesis by a circadian clock, the gating process involves an E box-mediated transcriptional activation of the adenyl cyclase gene. This regulates melatonin synthesis by regulating the expression of type 1 adenyl cyclase, and the synthesis of cAMP in photoreceptors (Fukuhara et al., 2004). Cyclic AMP signaling may play a key role in the input and output components of the central circadian axis, the retina, the SCN, and the pineal gland (Fukuhara et al., 2004). Although the studies cited above have been conducted in the chicken, several *in vivo* and *in vitro* studies have established that there is a circadian clock system in the mammalian eye independent from the SCN (Tosini et al., 2008). Besides the retina, it has been reported that both AA-NAT and HIOMT are present in other ocular structures such as lenses of rabbit and rat (Abe et al., 1999; Itoh et al., 2007).

3. MELATONIN RECEPTORS IN THE EYE

Since most of melatonin functions are attributed to its interaction with specific receptors, the study of the distribution of melatonin receptor subtypes in the eye assumes functional significance (Alarma-Estrany and Pintor, 2007). Immunocytochemical analysis of ocular tissues obtained from various species, including chickens, rats, and humans, shows that melatonin receptors type 1 and 2 (MT1 and MT2, formerly Mel_{1a} and Mel_{1b}, respectively) are localized in the cornea, choroid, sclera, retina, and retinal blood vessels (Ascher et al., 1995; Fujieda et al., 1999; Scher et al., 2002, 2003; Savaskan et al., 2002; Wiechmann et al., 2004; Rada and Wiechmann, 2006). In *Xenopus* eyes, MT1 have been described in the corneal epithelium, stroma, sclera, and endothelium (Wiechmann and Rada, 2003), suggesting melatonin's involvement in the differential regulation of growth and remodeling of the fibrous and cartilaginous scleral layers that affect eye size and refraction. On the other hand, the localization of melatonin receptors in the iris and ciliary processes could indicate that they may be involved in regulating IOP (Osborne et al., 1999). The presence of melatonin receptor Mel_{1c} in the non-pigmented epithelium of the chicken (Wiechmann and Wirsig-Wiechmann, 2001) suggests that melatonin may affect the rate of aqueous humor secretion by the ciliary epithelium and the circadian rhythm of IOP.

The Mel_{1c} receptor subtype was first cloned in the chicken (Liu et al., 1995), but has never been identified in mammals (Wiechmann and Summers, 2008). The three identified melatonin receptors, namely MT1, MT2 and Mel_{1c}, show different daily rhythms of protein expression in the retinal pigment epithelium, and choroid, with peak levels of MT1 and MT2 occurring during the night and peak levels of Mel_{1c} occurring during the day in the chick (Rada and Wiechmann, 2006). The presence of MT2 in *Xenopus* apical microvillar cell membrane but not on the basement membrane of the pigment epithelium supports the hypothesis that melatonin is involved in photoreceptor outer segment disk shedding and phagocytosis (Wiechmann and Rada, 2003; Wiechmann and Summers, 2008). It was originally reported that in the human retina, MT2 receptors are highly expressed compared to a relatively lower expression of MT1 receptors (Reppert et al., 1995), however a subsequent study reported similar levels of expression for both melatonin receptor types (Scher et al., 2002). MT1 receptors have been identified in RGCs and amacrine cells in rat and guinea pig (Fujieda et al., 1999, 2000). MT1 receptors are expressed in photoreceptors and other cell types of the human retina (Meyer et al., 2002; Scher et al., 2002, 2003). In humans, MT1 immunoreactivity was found in cell bodies along inner border of the inner nuclear layer, and in its outer border almost exclusively in horizontal cells, in cell bodies within the ganglion cell layer and in the inner segments of rod photoreceptors (Scher et al., 2002). In addition, about two thirds of CA1 and CA2 dopaminergic neurons exhibited MT1 immunolabeling. MT1 receptors were also identified in human and macaque AII amacrine cells, which are critical neurons in the rod pathway of the mammalian retina. The MT2 receptor is expressed in the sclera, lens, pigment epithelium, and neural retina of *Xenopus* eye (Wiechmann et al., 2004). In elderly humans, MT2 has recently been localized to ganglion and bipolar cells in the inner nuclear layer, to the inner segments of photoreceptors, and to cellular processes in inner and outer plexiform layers (Savaskan et al., 2007). The presence of melatonin receptors in multiple cell types suggests that melatonin could have multiple physiological functions in the retina. In human RGCs, MT1 receptors represent nearly 90% of the total number of melatonin receptors (Meyer et al., 2002). In one study, the MT1 receptor subtype expression in ganglion and amacrine cells from two patients with Alzheimer's disease was found to be significantly higher than in controls (Savaskan et al., 2002), suggesting that in this disease an up-regulation mechanism exists that evolves with very low melatonin levels (Ferrari et al., 2000). The MT1 receptor has been identified in the adventitial cells of retinal vessels, suggesting that melatonin could have an indirect action on vascular smooth muscle (Savaskan et al., 2002).

4. OCULAR FUNCTIONS OF MELATONIN

Systemic administration of melatonin has been found to produce significant changes in anterior and vitreous chamber depth, suggesting that melatonin may play a role in ocular growth and development (Rada and Wiechmann, 2006). Retinal melatonin acts as a neuromodulator that mediates dark adaptive regulation of retinomotor movements (Pierce and Besharse, 1985). The expression of MT1 receptors in most dopaminergic amacrine cells in human retina implicates melatonin in the modulation of dopaminergic function (Scher et al., 2003). Both dopamine and melatonin are key signaling agents in the regulation of retinal rhythmicity. These two substances are mutually inhibitory, acting as signals for day and night, respectively. It was demonstrated that picomolar concentrations of melatonin selectively inhibit the calcium-dependent release of dopamine from rabbit retina (Dubocovich, 1983). Moreover, experimental evidence which supports the model of mutual signaling between melatonin and dopamine has been provided by Doyle et al. (2002), who demonstrated that in C3H+/+ mice, which lack melatonin and show no circadian rhythmicity of dopamine content, the deficiency could be corrected by cyclical administration of melatonin. The action of melatonin on the rod pathway at the level of horizontal and amacrine cells has been proposed as a unique mechanism by which the retina adapts to low light intensities (Scher et al., 2002). A correlation between melatonin levels and the electroretinographic response has been shown in human studies which suggest that daily melatonin and electroretinogram cycling are associated (Rufiange et al., 2002).

5. OXIDATIVE STRESS IN GLAUCOMA AND THE ROLE OF MELATONIN AS AN ANTIOXIDANT

There is a considerable variety of free radicals in the organism that are produced as byproducts of molecular oxygen and that are able to exert extensive damage, particularly over time. Free radicals may destroy virtually any molecule they encounter. The retina is especially susceptible to oxidative stress because of its high oxygen consumption, its high proportion of polyunsaturated fatty acids, and its exposure to light. Among others, glutathione, and antioxidant enzymes such as superoxide dismutase (SOD), catalase, and glutathione peroxidase (GPX) provide a powerful antioxidant defense in the retina (Armstrong et al., 1981; Castorina et al., 1992; Ohta et al., 1996). However, despite having high levels of antioxidants, the retina is still susceptible to oxidative stress that has been observed in several retinal conditions (Wu et al., 1997; Tanito et al., 2002; van Reyk et al., 2003; Rajesh et al., 2003).

As for a link between oxidative damage and glaucoma, it has been reported that the level of lipid peroxidation products increases more than two fold and that the ocular antioxidant defense mechanism decreases in the anterior chamber humor of patients with advanced glaucoma (Kurysheva et al., 1996). Glaucoma is an optic neuropathy in which RGCs die individually or in small groups, typically over many years, and probably through an apoptotic process. The control of apoptosis is known to involve free radicals in several systems, including the retina (Giardino et al., 1998; Liversidge et al., 2002). In fact, antioxidant agents suppress retinal apoptosis induced by various insults, such as axotomy or photic injury (Tanito et al., 2002; Castagne et al., 2000). Oxidative damage may be considered as the cytopathic consequence of the generation of excess reactive oxygen species (ROS) beyond the cell's defensive capacity (Simonian and Coyle, 1996). Mounting evidence points to the involvement of these molecules in a broad range of neuropathologic disorders, probably by increasing the peroxidation of fatty acids or nucleic acids and protein cross-linking. SOD catalyzes the conversion of superoxide radicals (O_2^-) to hydrogen peroxide (H_2O_2), which is the first step in the metabolic defense against cellular oxidative stress. Although H_2O_2 is not a free radical, it is highly reactive, membrane permeable, and can be converted to highly reactive metabolites of oxygen such as hydroxyl radical. Under normal conditions, most of the H_2O_2 molecules generated by SOD are further metabolized to water by catalase and GPX. Thus, it is critical for the cellular survival that SOD activity should be coupled with similar GPX and catalase activities to safely detoxify H_2O_2. We have demonstrated that SOD and catalase (but not GPX) activities decrease in eyes with ocular hypertension induced by HA (Moreno et al, 2004). Although in normal physiological conditions, GPX seems to be more efficient compared to catalase in reducing organic peroxides (Holmgren, 1989; Sen, 1998),

Spector et al. (1996) reported that under conditions of knocked out or inhibited GPX, catalase is able to provide protection against oxidative stress. Furthermore, during acute oxidative stress, catalase induction has been shown to be many folds higher than the increase of GPX activity (Verkerk and Jongkind, 1992). It was demonstrated that especially in structures like the eye, catalase has a significant contribution to H_2O_2 detoxification. The inhibition of catalase activity in the eyes of rabbits increases H_2O_2 concentration 2.5-fold, which is not compensated by GPX activity (Ohta et al., 1996). Although the mechanism(s) involved in the changes of these retinal enzymatic activities from hypertensive eyes is not yet understood, it is highly probable that a decrease of SOD and catalase activities could provoke an imbalance of the endogenous antioxidant defense system. This hypothesis is strongly supported by a significant increase in retinal lipid peroxidation observed in the retinas from hypertensive eyes (Moreno et al., 2004).

The possibility that melatonin could detoxify highly reactive oxygen species was originally suggested by Ianas et al. (1991). Three years later, Reiter and coworkers (Reiter et al., 1994) using spin trapping and electron resonance spectroscopy, demonstrated melatonin's capacity to directly scavenge highly reactive hydroxyl radicals. Since then, several reports have shown that melatonin acts as a free radical scavenger and an efficient antioxidant (Hardeland et al., 1995; Reiter et al., 1997, 1998, 2000; Turjanski et al., 1998; Pandi-Perumal et al., 2006). Not only melatonin, but also several of its metabolites generated during its free radical scavenging action may act as antioxidants (Tan et al., 2007a). The kynurenic pathway of melatonin metabolism includes a series of radical scavengers with the possible sequence: Melatonin → cyclic 3-hydroxymelatonin → N^1-acetyl-N^2-formyl-5-methoxykynuramine (AFMK) → N^1-acetyl-5-methoxykynuramine (AMK). In the metabolic step from melatonin to AFMK, up to four free radicals can be consumed (Adler et al., 1997; Guenther et al., 2005; Hardeland, 2005; Tan et al., 2007a). Because of this pathway, melatonin's efficacy as an antioxidant is greatly increased. Melatonin has been shown to scavenge free radicals generated in mitochondria, reduce electron leakage from the respiratory complexes and improve ATP synthesis (Acuña-Castroviejo et al., 2003; León et al., 2005). Moreover, melatonin preserves mitochondrial glutathione levels, thereby enhancing the antioxidant potential (León et al., 2004). By scavenging free radicals, increasing the antioxidant defense system activity, and improving the electron transport chain at the mitochondrial level, melatonin is able to protect ocular tissues from oxidative damage (Siu et al., 2006; Lundmark et al., 2006).

It was demonstrated that the low affinity MT3 melatonin receptor binding site is identical with quinone reductase 2 (QR2) (Nosjean et al., 2000), and that melatonin inhibits the activity of this enzyme (Boutin et al., 2008; Calamini et al., 2008) and there is evidence that, contrary to previous belief (Tan et al., 2007b), QR2 is an activating enzyme (Long et al., 2002; Celli et al., 2006) since its deletion from living organisms leads to increased toxicity of quinones (Long et al., 2002). Thus, inhibition of QR2 could have antioxidant effects. Moreover, it was recently demonstrated that melatonin significantly increases SOD activity and GSH levels whereas it decreases retinal lipid peroxidation in the rat retina (Belforte et al., 2010). In the experimental model of glaucoma induced by injections of HA, a significant decrease in retinal melatonin levels was demonstrated (Moreno et al., 2004). Taking into account the conclusive evidences on the role of melatonin as antioxidant, together with the fall in retinal melatonin levels and with the decrease in the antioxidant defense system activity in hypertensive eyes, it is tempting to speculate about a causal relationship between these latter phenomena.

Whether retinal oxidative damage is involved in glaucomatous RGC death is far from being understood. Compared with other retinal cells, neonatal ganglion cells are remarkably resistant to cell death induced by superoxide anion, hydrogen peroxide, or hydroxyl radical, and it was postulated that this resistance may be mediated by the possession of sufficient constitutive levels of one or more peroxidases, probably catalase and/or GPX (Kortuem et al., 2000). Thus, it seems possible that a decrease of some of these enzymatic activities may overcome the capacity of these cells to resist oxidative damage. In summary, these results support the involvement of oxidative stress in glaucomatous damage. Thus, manipulation of intracellular redox status using antioxidants such as melatonin may be a new therapeutic tool to prevent glaucomatous cell death.

6. NITROSATIVE STRESS IN GLAUCOMA AND ANTI-NITRIDERGIC EFFECTS OF MELATONIN

NO is a ubiquitous signaling molecule that participates in a variety of cellular functions. However, in concert with reactive oxygen species, NO can be transformed into a highly potent and effective cytotoxic entity of pathophysiological significance. NO may also signal through the interaction with reduced cysteines of proteins changing protein function (Martinez-Ruiz and Lamas, 2004). As an intracellular signaling molecule, NO modulates the activity of various proteins that contribute to apoptosis (Melino et al., 1997). Furthermore, it was demonstrated that an extracellular proteolytic pathway in the retina contributes to RGC death *via* NO-activated metalloproteinase-9 (Manabe et al., 2005). Several lines of evidence support a link between NO and glaucoma. In that sense, an increased presence of neuronal NOS (NOS-1 or nNOS) and inducible NOS (NOS-2 or iNOS), was reported in astrocytes of the lamina cribrosa and ONH of patients with POAG (Neufeld et al.,1997; Liu and Neufeld, 2000). In rats whose extraocular veins were cauterized to produce chronic ocular hypertension and retinal damage, expression of NOS-2 but not NOS-1 increases in ONH astrocytes (Liu and Neufeld, 2003). Moreover, elevation of hydrostatic pressure *in vitro* upregulates the expression of NOS-2 in human astrocytes derived from the ONH (Liu and Neufeld, 2001). Most important, inhibition of NOS-2 by aminoguanidine or L-N(6)-(1-iminoethyl)lysine 5-tetrazole amide protects against RGC loss in the rat cautery model of glaucoma (Neufeld, 2004; Neufeld et al., 1999). These data support that activation of NOS, especially NOS-2, may play a significant role in glaucomatous optic neuropathy. However, later on, Pang et al. (2005) showed that chronically elevated IOP in the rat induced by episcleral injection of hypertonic saline does not increase NOS-2 immunoreactivity in the optic nerve, ONH, or ganglion cell layer. Moreover, retinal and ONH NOS-2 mRNA levels did not correlate with either IOP level or severity of optic nerve injury. In addition, there was no difference in NOS-2 immunoreactivity in the optic nerve or ONH between POAG and nonglaucomatous eyes (Pang et al., 2005), and aminoguanidine treatment did not affect the development of pressure-induced optic neuropathy in rats (Pang et al., 2005). A significant activation of the retinal nitridergic pathway was described in the experimental model of glaucoma induced by intracameral injections of HA (Belforte et al., 2007). Despite that other studies (mostly based on Western blotting or immunohistochemical analysis) previously addressed the issue of NO involvement in human or experimental glaucoma, they did not assessed changes in the functional capacity of the retinal nitridergic pathway. Although no changes in the levels of NOS isoforms were observed in HA-treated eyes, a significant increase of the retinal arginine to citrulline conversion was demonstrated in HA-injected eyes (Belforte et al., 2007). The intracellular events triggered by ocular hypertension that could explain the increase in retinal NOS activity, remain to be established. However, since glutamate acting through NMDA receptors is one of the most conspicuous activators of NOS-1 activity, the raise in glutamate synaptic levels in HA-treated eyes (as discussed below) could account for it. In this sense, it was shown that RGCs in the nNOS-deficient mouse were relatively resistant to NMDA, while damage in the retina of the endothelial NOS-deficient mouse was not distinguishable from that observed in control animals (Vorwerk et al., 1997). Moreover, it was demonstrated that intravitreal injection of NMDA in rats induces accumulation of nitrite/nitrate (El-Remessy et al., 2003).

A significant increase in the retinal uptake of L-arginine (a NOS substrate) was demonstrated in HA-treated eyes. Purified NOS from different sources has been reported to have a low half-saturating L-arginine concentration (EC_{50}) ~ 10 μM. Since high levels of intracellular L-arginine ranging from 0.1 - 1 mM have been measured in many systems (Block et al., 1995), it is expected that endogenous L-arginine would support maximal activation of NOS. However, a number of *in vivo* and *in vitro* studies indicate that NO production under physiological conditions can be increased by extracellular L-arginine, despite saturating intracellular L-arginine concentrations. This has been termed "the arginine paradox" (Kurz and Harrison, 1997). One possible explanation could be that intracellular L-arginine is sequestered in one or more pools that are poorly, if at all, accessible to NOS, whereas extracellular L-arginine transported into the cells is preferentially delivered to NO biosynthesis (Kurz and Harrison, 1997). Accordingly, it was demonstrated that L-arginine availability controls NMDA-induced NO synthesis in the rat central nervous system (Grima et al., 1998). Therefore, it seems likely that to induce the activation of NOS, an obligatory influx of L-arginine is required. The coordination between NOS activity and L-arginine uptake has been demonstrated in several systems such as rat brain (Stevens et al., 1996), and diabetic rat retina (do Carmo et al., 1998). A similar coordination between NO biosynthesis and intracellular L-arginine availability seems to occur in hypertensive eyes. It was demonstrated that activation of NMDA receptors in cultured retinal cells promotes an increase of the intracellular L-arginine pool available for NO synthesis (Cossenza et al., 2006). This way, the increase in both NOS activity and L-arginine influx, could be triggered by higher levels of synaptic glutamate levels.

Four amino acid transport systems (denoted by y^+, $b^{o,+}$, $B^{o,+}$ or y^+L) have been defined on the basis of substrate specificity and sodium dependence (for review, see Devés and Boyd, 1998). Only one of them (y^+) is selective for cationic amino acids and sodium-independent. It was demonstrated that the uptake of L-arginine in retinas from rats and hamsters occurs through a transporter resembling the y^+ system (Carmo et al., 1999; Sáenz et al., 2002a). This transport system encompasses three homologous proteins (named cationic amino acid transporter (CAT)-1, CAT-2, and CAT-3) that have been characterized in several tissues. RT-PCR analysis using primers for the aforementioned isoforms demonstrated an increase of mRNAs for both CAT-1 and CAT-2 in retinas from hypertensive eyes, suggesting that ocular hypertension could induce an upregulation of L-arginine transporters (Belforte et al., 2007).

It was demonstrated that melatonin inhibits the nitridergic pathway activity in the golden hamster (Sáenz et al., 2002b) and rat retina (Belforte et al., 2010). Melatonin significantly decreases retinal NOS activity and L-arginine uptake, and inhibits the accumulation of cGMP induced by both L-arginine and a NO donor. The inhibitory effect of melatonin on retinal NOS activity is consistent with the previously described effect of melatonin on this enzyme from other neural structures (Bettahi et al., 1996; Pozo et al., 1997; León et al., 1998). However, while the effect of melatonin in those tissues was evident up to 1 nM, a much higher sensitivity to the methoxyindole was evident in the hamster retina, since it is effective even at 1 pM, suggesting that the retinal nitridergic pathway is regulated by physiological concentrations of melatonin (Sáenz et al., 2002b). In addition to inhibiting NOS activity, melatonin is able to directly scavenge NO, generating at least one stable product, i.e., N-nitrosomelatonin (Turjanski, et al., 2000). Moreover, melatonin reduces NO-induced lipid peroxidation in rat retinal homogenates and ileum tissue sections (Siu et al., 1999; Cuzzocrea et al., 2000). Taken together, these results indicate that melatonin modulates the nitridergic pathway in an opposite way to that induced by ocular hypertension, as shown in Figure 1.

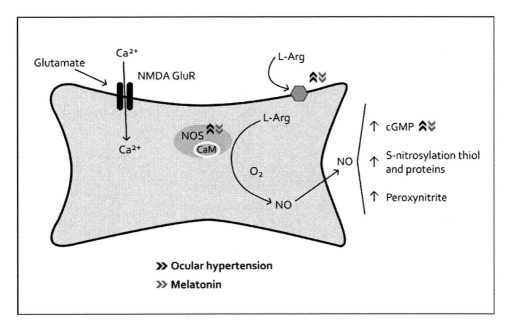

Figure 1. Schematic representation of the retinal nitridergic pathway and its modulation by melatonin and ocular hypertension. Weekly injections of HA induces an increase in retinal NOS activity and L-arginine uptake, whereas melatonin regulates this parameters in an opposite way. Positive effects are noted as ⋀, whereas ⋁ indicates negative modulations.

7. EXCITOTOXICITY IN GLAUCOMA AND THE EFFECT OF MELATONIN ON GLUTAMATE CLEARANCE

Glutamate is the main excitatory neurotransmitter in the retina, but it is toxic when present in excessive amounts. Retinal tissue is in fact, an established paradigm for glutamate neurotoxicity for several reasons: (i) insult leads to accumulation of relatively high levels of glutamate in the extracellular fluid (Louzada-Junior et al., 1992), (ii) administration of glutamate leads to neuronal cell death (David et al., 1988); and (iii) glutamate receptor antagonists can protect against neuronal degeneration (Mosinger et al., 1991). Thus, an appropriate clearance of synaptic glutamate is required for the normal function of retinal excitatory synapses and for prevention of neurotoxicity. Glial cells, mainly astrocytes and Müller glia, surround glutamatergic synapses, and express glutamate transporters and the glutamate-metabolizing enzyme, glutamine synthetase (GS) (Riepe and Norenburg, 1977; Sarthy and Lam, 1978). Glutamate is transported into glial cells and amidated by GS to the non-toxic aminoacid glutamine. Glutamine is then released by the glial cells and taken up by neurons, where it is hydrolyzed by glutaminase to form glutamate again, completing the retinal glutamate/glutamine cycle (Figure 2) (Thoreson and Witkovsky, 1999; Poitry et al., 2000). In this way, the neurotransmitter pool is replenished and glutamate neurotoxicity is prevented. Glutamatergic injury has been proposed to contribute to the RGC death in glaucoma. This hypothesis is supported by the demonstration that vitreal glutamate is elevated in glaucomatous dogs (Brooks et al., 1997), and quail with congenital glaucoma (Dkhissi et al., 1999). In addition, high glutamine levels were been found in retinal Müller cells of glaucomatous rat eyes (Shen et al., 2004). In contrast, other authors showed no significant elevation of glutamate in the vitreous of patients with glaucoma (Honkanen et al., 2003), or in rats (Levkovitch-Verbin et al., 2002), and monkeys with experimental glaucoma (Carter-Dawson et al., 2002; Wamsley et al., 2005). In any case, it seems limited a viewpoint to assume that high levels of glutamate in the vitreous are a necessary condition for excitotoxicity to be involved in glaucomatous neuropathy. The local concentration of glutamate at the membrane receptors of RGCs is the important issue for toxicity.

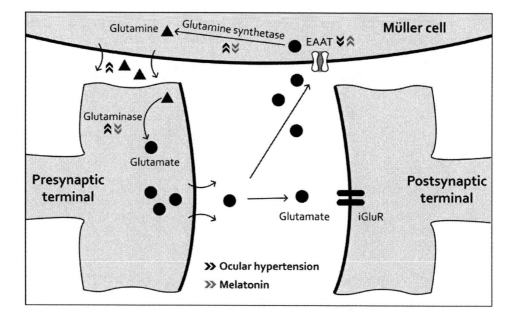

Figure 2. Schematic representation of the retinal glutamate/glutamine cycle, and its modulation by melatonin. As shown, ocular hypertension decreases glutamate uptake and GS activity, and increases glutamine uptake and release, and glutaminase activity. On the other hand, melatonin increases glutamate uptake, glutamate release, GS activity, and glutamine uptake, whereas it decreases glutaminase activity. Positive effects are noted as ⋀, whereas ⋁ indicates negative modulations.

This could be very different from the level in samples of vitreous. Vitreous humor must be removed for experimental measurement by a process that inevitably disturbs its state before removal. These manipulations could themselves alter the measured amount of glutamate. At present, there are no available tools to directly assess retinal glutamate synaptic concentrations *in vivo*. However, glutamate synaptic concentrations could be estimated by studying the retinal mechanisms that regulate glutamate clearance and recycling. We have demonstrated a significant alteration of the retinal glutamate/glutamine cycle activity in rats exposed to experimentally elevated IOP (Moreno et al., 2005a). Since no enzymes exist extracellularly that degrade glutamate, glutamate transporters are responsible for maintaining low synaptic glutamate concentrations. Retinal glutamate uptake significantly decreases in HA-treated eyes. In agreement, a significant reduction in the amount of the main retinal glutamate transporter (excitatory amino acid transporter type 1, (EAAT-1)) assessed by Western blot analysis in a rat glaucoma model (Martin et al., 2002), and a downregulation of this transporter in retinal Müller cells from glaucoma patients (Naskar et al., 2000) were demonstrated. While these studies did not assess changes in the functional capacity of glutamate transporters, our results demonstrated a removing glutamate disability in retinas from hypertensive eyes. The synaptically released glutamate is taken up into glial cells, where GS converts it into glutamine. Since Müller cells rapidly convert glutamate to glutamine, the driving force for glutamate uptake would be stronger in these cells than in neurons, which have much higher intracellular free glutamate concentrations (Pow and Robinson, 1994). In fact, although glutamate uptake is controlled by the expression and post-translational modifications, physiological measurements suggest that glutamate uptake may also depend on its metabolism (Gegelashvili and Schousboe, 1998; Tanaka, 2000). Indeed, an increase in internal glutamate concentrations significantly slows down the net transport of glutamate, and it was suggested that instantaneous intracellular glutamate metabolism may be needed for efficient glutamate clearance of the extracellular milieu (Attwell et al., 1993; Otis and Jahr, 1998). Thus, a decrease in GS activity could account for a decrease in glutamate uptake. Glutamine is released from Müller cells and could be a precursor for neuronal glutamate synthesis. The increase in the basal release and the uptake of glutamine in HA-treated eyes could provoke a raise in the availability of substratum for glutamate synthesis. Moreover, this increase in glutamate production could be further potentiated by the augment of GS. Decreasing the levels of expression of the EAAT1 increases vitreal glutamate, and is toxic to RGCs (Vorwerk et al., 2000). Thus, the decrease in glutamate influx could provoke an increase in synaptic glutamate levels. In addition, a decrease of GS activity, as well as in increase in glutaminase activity in retinas form hypertensive eyes could contribute synergically and/or redundantly to an excessive increase in synaptic glutamate levels (Moreno et al., 2005a).

Nanomolar concentrations of melatonin significantly modulate the glutamate/glutamine cycle activity in the golden hamster (Sáenz et al., 2004) and rat retina (Belforte et al., 2010). In that sense, it was demonstrated that low concentrations of melatonin significantly increase retinal glutamate uptake and GS activity, and decrease glutaminase activity. This way, melatonin may contribute to the conversion of glutamate to glutamine through a possibly redundant mechanism. The physiological consequences of a modulation by melatonin of the retinal glutamate/glutamine cycle are yet to be determined, although this effect could provide new insights into the neuroprotective potential of melatonin. In that respect, it was demonstrated that an increase in GS provides neuroprotection in experimental models of neurodegeneration (Gorovits et al., 1997; Heidinger et al., 1999). Induction of GS *in vivo* or *in vitro* by glucocorticoids was clearly demonstrated in different tissues, including the retina

(Sarkar and Chaudhury, 1983; Patel et al., 1983). Physiological levels of glucocorticoids regulate GS expression by stimulating the gene transcription. This effect of glucocorticoids has been associated to their ability to protect against neuronal degeneration (Gorovits et al., 1997), as shown in animal models of brain injury (Hall, 1985), as well as after retinal photic injury (Rosner et al., 1992). However, since induction of GS expression by glucocorticoids takes about 24 h, there are some potential weaknesses in glucocorticoid treatment. In contrast, since the effect of melatonin is much faster (in the range of minutes) a treatment with the methoxyindole may circumvent this obstacle. Furthermore, this beneficial effect of melatonin may be further improved by its effect on glutamate uptake, and glutaminase activity. In summary, these findings suggest that a treatment with melatonin could be considered as a new approach to handling glutamate-mediated neuronal degeneration, such as that induced by glaucoma (Figure 2).

8. GABAergic Dysfunction in Glaucoma and the Effect of Melatonin on the Retinal GABAergic System

The neurochemical organization maintained throughout vertebrate retinas is that glutamate is the neurotransmitter in the photoreceptor cell→ bipolar cell→ ganglion cell chain, whereas GABA is used by numerous horizontal and amacrine cells in the lateral pathway, modulating neural transmission in both synaptic layers (Kalloniatis and Tomisich, 1999; Yang, 2004). Retinal output neurons communicate by liberating glutamate, while tonically or phasically active inhibitory neurons (mostly GABAergic) modulate the passage of information, offering resistance against which the firing tendencies, which results in variable levels of neural activity. The prevailing view is that the balance between excitatory and inhibitory signaling plays a pivotal role in mechanisms underlying the modulation and maintenance of a variety of retinal functions and sensory information encoding. In fact, the loss of this balance could provoke cell death. Despite the putative involvement of glutamate in glaucomatous cell death previously discussed, and the key role of GABA in retinal function, the GABAergic activity was not extensively examined in experimental models of glaucoma. Recently, a significant dysfunction of the retinal GABAergic system was demonstrated in rats exposed to experimentally elevated IOP (Moreno et al., 2008). These results indicate that retinal GABA steady state concentrations, GABA turnover rate, glutamic acid decarboxylase (GAD) activity, GABA transporters (GATs), and GABA receptors are susceptible to ocular hypertension (Figure 3).

Retinal GABA release involves two distinct components; one requires extracellular calcium, while the other is calcium-independent and involves reversal of the operating direction of a high affinity GABA carrier (Schwartz, 1987). Although differences in retinal GABA release were observed among species, glutamate induces GABA release mostly *via* a Ca^{2+}-independent Na^+-dependent carrier mechanism, while high K^+-induced GABA release is partially calcium-dependent (do Nascimento et al., 1998; López-Costa et al., 1999; Andrade da Costa et al., 2000). Retinal GABA release induced by both stimuli significantly decreases in the retina from HA-injected eyes, supporting that ocular hypertension affects the carrier-mediated component. As significant changes in GABA influx is also observed in HA-treated eyes (Moreno et al., 2008), ocular hypertension may influence the preferred direction of GABA transporters provoking a switch from release to uptake. Indeed, since GAD activity significantly decreases in HA-treated eyes, the driving force for GABA uptake would be stronger in cells with lower intracellular GABA concentrations, favoring its uptake over its release.

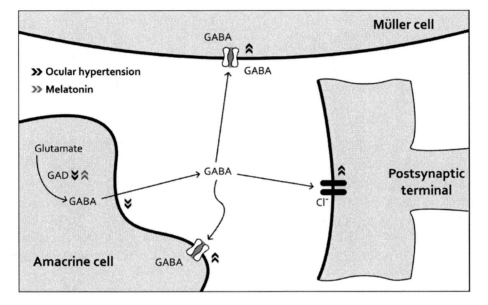

Figure 3. Schematic representation of the modulation of the retinal GABAergic system activity by ocular hypertension and melatonin. Ocular hypertension significantly increases GABA uptake and decreases GABA turnover rate, GAD activity and GABA release. In control retinas, melatonin increases GABA turnover rate and GAD activity. Positive effects are noted as ⋀, whereas ⋁ indicates negative modulations.

GATs in cells surrounding the release site are responsible for terminating GABA signals within the retina (Gadea and López-Colomé, 2001). GATs were mainly localized in amacrine, displaced amacrine, RGCs, and Müller cells (Honda et al., 1995; Johnson et al., 1996). GABA uptake is significantly higher in retinas from eyes injected with HA (Figure 3), which could contribute synergically and/or redundantly to a significant decrease of synaptic GABA levels in retinas exposed to ocular hypertension.

To our knowledge, there is no other retinal pathological condition in which a GABAergic deficit has been previously described. However, a decrease in GABAergic neurotransmission has been implicated in the pathophysiology of several central nervous system disorders, particularly in epilepsy. In this case, excessive glutamate-mediated neurotransmission and impaired GABA-mediated inhibition, among other mechanisms, may trigger a cascade of events leading to neuronal damage and cell death. Excitotoxicity is a common pathogenetic mechanism in neurodegenerative diseases, including probably glaucoma, which may result from the failure of normal compensatory antiexcitatory mechanisms, necessary to maintain cellular homeostasis. An abnormal glutamate outflow may play a crucial role in triggering cellular events leading to excitotoxic neuronal death. Reduced synaptic inhibition as a result of a GABAergic dysfunction could be one of the major causes for this imbalance. In this way, ocular hypertension may greatly shift the balance between retinal excitation and inhibition.

As mentioned before, we have demonstrated an increase in glutamate synaptic concentrations in retinas from eyes injected with HA (Moreno et al., 2005a). Since an increase in synaptic glutamate or its residence time in the synaptic region is toxic to RGCs (Kawasaki et al., 2000; Nucci et al., 2005), the decrease in GABAergic activity could make worse glutamate toxicity. In this way, the deficit in GABAergic activity could contribute to glaucomatous neuropathy.

It was demonstrated that melatonin increases retinal GABA levels, as shown by its effect on GABA turnover rate and GAD activity (Belforte et al., 2010). The effect of melatonin on the GABAergic activity seems not to be exclusive for the retina, since it was previously demonstrated that melatonin increases GABA turnover rate and GAD activity in rat hypothalamus, cerebellum, and cerebral cortex (Rosenstein and Cardinali, 1986; Rosenstein et al., 1989). These results indicate that glaucomatous damage may involve a decrease in GABA synaptic levels, which can be restored by a treatment with melatonin (Figure 3).

9. EFFECT OF MELATONIN ON GLAUCOMATOUS DAMAGE

Data previously mentioned indicate that melatonin is able to impair glutamate neurotoxicity, decrease NO levels, increase GABA concentrations, and reduce oxidative stress, and that an increase in glutamate and NO levels, a decrease in the GABAergic activity, and oxidative damage could be involved in glaucomatous neuropathy. Thus, it seems likely that melatonin could have a beneficial effect against glaucoma. This hypothesis was recently analyzed in the glaucoma model induced by HA injections (Belforte et al., 2010). For this purpose, a pellet of melatonin was implanted subcutaneously 24 h before the first injection of HA. Melatonin, which did not affect IOP, prevented the effect of ocular hypertension on retinal function (assessed by electroretinography), and diminished the vulnerability of RGCs to the deleterious effects of ocular hypertension (Belforte et al., 2010). Although melatonin conferred neuroprotection in the experimental model of glaucoma induced by HA, the translational relevance of this result is limited by the fact that melatonin was administered before the induction of ocular hypertension (e.g. 24 h before the first injection of HA). Human open angle glaucoma is a progressive optic neuropathy. In agreement, different stages were identified in the experimental model of glaucoma induced by HA, showing the following characteristics: i) 3 weeks of ocular hypertension: increase in glutamate and NO levels, decrease in GABA levels, and incipient oxidative stress, without changes in the ERG and retinal morphology (e.g. *asymptomatic ocular hypertension*); ii) 6 weeks of ocular hypertension: increase in NO levels, higher oxidative stress, and decrease in the ERG without histological changes (e.g. *moderated glaucoma*); and iii) 10 weeks of ocular hypertension: higher oxidative stress, further decrease in the ERG (vs. 6 weeks), and loss of RGCs and optic nerve fibers (e.g. *advanced glaucoma*) (Moreno et al., 2005b). To analyze the therapeutic effect, a pellet of melatonin was implanted at 6 weeks of ocular hypertension, a time point in which functional alterations are already evident, and the results indicate that the delayed treatment with melatonin of eyes with ocular hypertension resulted in similar protection when compared with eyes treated from the onset of ocular hypertension. We do not have any clear explanation for these results. We have shown that an increase in synaptic glutamate concentrations (Moreno et al., 2005a) and NO production (Belforte et al., 2007), as well as a GABAergic dysfunction (Moreno et al., 2008) occur mostly prior to 6 weeks of ocular hypertension induced by HA. Based on these results, it seems possible that alterations in glutamate, NO, and GABA may trigger an initial insult responsible for initiation of damage that is followed by a slower secondary degeneration that ultimately results in cell death. In that sense, we showed that oxidative stress is a longer lasting phenomenon which can be observed even at 10 weeks of ocular hypertension (Moreno et al., 2004). In this scenario, the preventive effect of melatonin (shown by the administration of melatonin before the first injection of HA) could be explained by the decrease in glutamate and NO levels and an increase in GABA concentrations, while its therapeutic effect (shown by the administration of melatonin at 6 weeks of ocular hypertension) can be explained essentially by its antioxidant effect. In this context, the fact that melatonin was similarly effective in the chronically treated animals and the delayed treatment, could support the hypothesis that in both cases melatonin is able to reverse oxidative damage which could be a key factor in glaucomatous dysfunction and cell death.

Neuroprotection in glaucoma implies the use of drugs or chemicals to slow down whatever causes loss of vision (RGC death), without influencing IOP. In order to be effective, a neuroprotectant must reach the ONH and/or RGCs and will therefore probably have to be taken orally (Osborne et al., 1999). Because it will reach other parts of the body, any side-effect of an appropriate neuroprotectant must be reduced to a minimum. Melatonin, a very safe compound for human use, is highly lipophilic and readily diffuses into tissues. In fact, subcutaneously administered, melatonin reaches the retina (Sande et al., 2008), increasing the local levels of the methoxyindole. RGCs are induced to die by different triggers in glaucoma, suggesting that neuroprotectants with multiple modes of actions are likely be effective in the therapeutic management of glaucoma (Marcic et al., 2003). Besides the mechanisms already described, there are other beneficial mechanisms of melatonin for glaucoma treatment. Several lines of evidence support that the obstruction of retrograde transport at the ONH results in the deprivation of neurotrophic support to RGCs, leading to apoptotic cell death in glaucoma (Tang et al., 2006). An important corollary to this concept is the implication that appropriate enhancement of neurotrophic support will prolong the survival of injured RGCs. Of particular importance is the fact that brain-derived neurotrophic factor (BDNF) not only promotes RGC survival following damage to the optic nerve, but also helps to preserve the structural integrity of the surviving neurons, which in turn results in enhanced visual function (Weber et al., 2008). As for the link between melatonin and neurotrophins, it has been suggested that melatonin may participate in neurodevelopment and in the regulation of neurotrophic factors (Niles et al, 2004; Jimenez et al., 2007). *In vitro*, melatonin promotes the viability and neuronal differentiation of neural stem cells and increases their production of BDNF (Kong et al., 2008). Moreover, ramelteon (a melatonin receptor agonist) is capable of increasing BDNF protein in primary cultures of cerebellar granule cells (Imbesi et al, 2008). In addition to ocular hypertension, the majority of glaucoma patients show signs of reduced ocular blood flow as well as ischemic signs in the eye, supporting that hemodynamic factors are involved as well in glaucomatous neuropathy. In this sense, it was shown that melatonin could increase the survival rate and rescue and restore injured RGCs in an experimental model of ischemia/reperfusion in rats (Tang et al., 2006), and it counteracts ischemia induced apoptosis in human retinal pigment epithelial cells (Osborne et al., 1998). Finally, while the cellular mechanisms involved in RGC loss observed in glaucomatous neuropathy are based on an apoptosis phenomenon, melatonin was shown to have antiapoptotic properties acting through several mechanisms, such as reduction of caspases, cytochrome c release, and modulation of Bcl-2 and Bax genes, among others. Taking together, these data indicate that melatonin seems to fulfill all the requirements to be considered a promissory neuroprotectant for glaucoma treatment. Alone or combined with an ocular hypotensive therapy, a treatment with melatonin, a very safe compound for human use, could be a new therapeutic tool helping the challenge faced by ophthalmologists treating glaucoma.

REFERENCES

Abe, M., Itoh, M. T., Miyata, M., Ishikawa, S. and Sumi, Y. (1999). Detection of melatonin, its precursors and related enzyme activities in rabbit lens. *Experimental Eye Research*, 68, 255-262.

Acuña-Castroviejo, D., Escames, G., Leon, J., Carazo, A. and Khaldy, H. (2003). Mitochondrial regulation by melatonin and its metabolites. *Advances in Experimental Medicine and Biology*, 527, 549-557.

Adler, L. J., Gyulai, F. E., Diehl, D. J., Mintun, M. A., Winter, P. M. and Firestone, L. L. (1997). Regional brain activity changes associated with fentanyl analgesia elucidated by positron emission tomography. *Anesthesia and Analgesia*, 84, 120-126.

Alarma-Estrany, P. and Pintor, J. (2007). Melatonin receptors in the eye: location, second messengers and role in ocular physiology. *Pharmacology and Therapeutics*, 113, 507-522.

Alonso-Gómez, A. L. and Iuvone, P. M. (1995). Melatonin biosynthesis in cultured chick retinal photoreceptor cells: calcium and cyclic AMP protect serotonin N-acetyltransferase from inactivation in cycloheximide-treated cells. *Journal of Neurochemistry*, 65, 1054-1060.

Andrade da Costa, B. L., de Mello, F. G. and Hokoc, J. N. (2000). Transporter mediated GABA release induced by excitatory amino acid agonist is associated with GAD-67 but not GAD-65 immunoreactive cells of the primate retina. *Brain Research*, 863, 132-142.

Armstrong, D., Santangelo, G. and Connole, E. (1981). The distribution of peroxide regulating enzymes in the canine eye. *Current Eye Research*, 1, 225-242.

Ascher, J. A., Cole, J. O., Colin, J. N., Feighner, J. P., Ferris, R. M., Fibiger, H. C., Golden, R. N., Martin, P., Potter, W. Z. and Richelson, E. (1995). Bupropion: a review of its mechanism of antidepressant activity. *Journal of Clinical Psychiatry*, 56, 395-401.

Aslan, M., Cort, A. and Yucel, I. (2008) Oxidative and nitrative stress markers in glaucoma. *Free Radical Biology and Medicine*, 45, 367-376.

Attwell, D., Barbour, B. and Szatkowski, M. (1993). Nonvesicular release of neurotransmitter. *Neuron*, 11, 401-407.

Axelrod, J. (1974). The pineal gland: a neurochemical transducer. Science, 184, 1341-1348.

Bailey, M. J., Chong, N. W., Xiong, J. and Cassone, V. M. (2002). Chickens' Cry2: molecular analysis of an avian cryptochrome in retinal and pineal photoreceptors. *FEBS Letters,* 513, 169-174.

Belforte, N., Moreno, M. C., Cymeryng, C., Bordone, M., Keller Sarmiento, M. I. and Rosenstein, R. E. (2007). Effect of ocular hypertension on retinal nitridergic pathway activity. *Investigative Ophthalmology and Visual Science*, 48, 2127-2133.

Belforte, N. A., Moreno, M. C., de Zavalía, N., Sande, P. H., Chianelli, M. S., Keller Sarmiento, M. I. and Rosenstein, R. E. (2010). Melatonin: a novel neuroprotectant for the treatment of glaucoma. *Journal of Pineal Research*, 48, 353-364.

Benozzi, J., Nahum, L. P., Campanelli, J. L. and Rosenstein, R. E. (2002). Effect of hyaluronic acid on intraocular pressure in rats. *Investigative Ophthalmology and Visual Science*, 43, 2196-2200.

Bernard, M., Guerlotte, J., Greve, P., Grechez-Cassiau, A., Iuvone, M. P., Zatz, M., Chong, N. W., Klein, D. C. and Voisin, P. (1999). Melatonin synthesis pathway: circadian regulation of the genes encoding the key enzymes in the chicken pineal gland and retina. *Reproduction, Nutrition, Development*, 39, 325-334.

Bettahi, I., Pozo, D., Osuna, C., Reiter, R. J., Acuña-Castroviejo, D. and Guerrero, J. M. (1996). Melatonin reduces nitric oxide synthase activity in rat hypothalamus. *Journal of Pineal Research*, 20, 205-210.

Block, E.R., Herrera, H. and Couch, M. (1995). Hypoxia inhibits L-arginine uptake by pulmonary artery endothelial cells. *American Journal of Physiology*, 269, L574-L580.

Boutin, J. A., Marcheteau, E., Hennig, P., Moulharat, N., Berger, S., Delagrange, P., Bouchet, J. P. and Ferry, G. (2008). MT3/QR2 melatonin binding site does not use melatonin as a substrate or a co-substrate. *Journal of Pineal Research*, 45, 524-531.

Brooks, D. E., Garcia, G. A., Dreyer, E. B., Zurakowski, D. and Franco-Bourland, R. E. (1997). Vitreous body glutamate concentration in dogs with glaucoma. *American Journal of Veterinary Research*, 58, 864-867.

Cahill,G. M. and Besharse, J. C. (1993). Circadian clock functions localized in xenopus retinal photoreceptors. *Neuron*, 10, 573-577.

Calamini, B., Santarsiero, B. D., Boutin, J. A. and Mesecar, A. D. (2008). Kinetic, thermodynamic and X-ray structural insights into the interaction of melatonin and analogues with quinone reductase 2. *The Biochemical Journal*, 413, 81-91.

Cardinali, D. P. and Rosner, J. M. (1971a). Metabolism of serotonin by the rat retina in vitro. *Journal of Neurochemistry*, 18, 1769-1770.

Cardinali, D. P. and Rosner, J. M. (1971b). Retinal localization of the hydroxyindole-0-methyl transferase (HIOMT) in the rat. *Endocrinology*, 89, 301-303.

Carmo, A., Cunha-Vaz, J. G., Carvalho, A. P. and Lopes, M. C. (1999). L-arginine transport in retinas from streptozotocin diabetic rats: correlation with the level of IL-1 beta and NO synthase activity. *Vision Research*, 39, 3817-3823.

Carter-Dawson, L., Crawford, M. L., Harwerth, R. S., Smith, E. L. 3rd, Feldman, R. and Shen, F. F. (2002). Vitreal glutamate concentration in monkeys with experimental glaucoma. *Investigative Ophthalmology and Visual Science*, 43, 2633-2637.

Castagne, V. and Clarke, P. G. (2000). Neuroprotective effects of a new glutathione peroxidase mimetic on neurons of the chick embryo's retina. *Journal of Neuroscience Research*, 59, 497-503.

Castorina, C., Campisi, A., Di Giacomo, C., Sorrenti, V., Russo, A. and Vanella, A. (1992). Lipid peroxidation and antioxidant enzymatic systems in rat retina as a function of age. *Neurochemical Research*, 17, 599-604.

Celli, C. M., Tran, N., Knox, R. and Jaiswal, A. K. (2006). NRH:quinone oxidoreductase 2 (NQO2) catalyzes metabolic activation of quinones and anti-tumor drugs. *Biochemical Pharmacology*, 72, 366-376.

Coon, S. L., Del, O. E., Young, W. S., III and Klein, D. C. (2002). Melatonin synthesis enzymes in Macaca mulatta: focus on arylalkylamine N-acetyltransferase (EC 2.3.1.87). *The Journal of Clinical Endocrinology and Metabolism*, 87, 4699-4706.

Coon, S. L., Mazuruk, K., Bernard, M., Roseboom, P. H., Klein, D. C. and Rodriguez, I. R. (1996). The human serotonin N-acetyltransferase (EC 2.3.1.87) gene (AANAT): structure, chromosomal localization, and tissue expression. *Genomics, 34*, 76-84.

Cossenza, M., Cadilhe, D.V., Coutinho, R. N. and Paes-de-Carvalho, R. (2006). Inhibition of protein synthesis by activation of NMDA receptors in cultured retinal cells: a new mechanism for the regulation of nitric oxide production. *Journal of Neurochemistry*, 97, 1481-1493.

Cuzzocrea, S., Costantino, G., Mazzon, E., Micali, A., De Sarro, A. and Caputi, A. P. (2000). Beneficial effects of melatonin in a rat model of splanchnic artery occlusion and reperfusion. *Journal of Pineal Research*, 28, 52-63.

David, P., Lusky, M. and Teichberg, V. I. (1988). Involvement of excitatory neurotransmitters in the damage produced in chick embryo retinas by anoxia and extracellular high potassium. *Experimental Eye Research*, 46, 657-662.

Devés, R. and Boyd, C. A. (1998). Transporters for cationic amino acids in animal cells: discovery, structure, and function. *Physiological Reviews*, 78, 487-545.

Dkhissi, O., Chanut, E., Wasowicz, M., Savoldelli, M., Nguyen-Legros, J., Minvielle, F. and Versaux-Botteri,C. (1999). Retinal TUNEL-positive cells and high glutamate levels in vitreous humor of mutant quail with a glaucoma-like disorder. *Investigative Ophthalmology and Visual Science*, 409, 90-95.

do Carmo, A., Lopes, C., Santos, M., Proença, R., Cunha-Vaz, J. and Carvalho AP. (1998). Nitric oxide synthase activity and L-arginine metabolism in the retinas from streptozotocin-induced diabetic rats. *General Pharmacology*, 30, 319-324.

do Nascimento, J. L., Ventura, A. L. and Paes de Carvalho, R. (1998). Veratridineand glutamate-induced release of [3H]-GABA from cultured chick retina cells: possible involvement of a GAT-1-like subtype of GABA transporter. *Brain Research*, 798, 217–222.

Doyle, S. E., Grace, M. S., McIvor, W. and Menaker, M. (2002). Circadian rhythms of dopamine in mouse retina: the role of melatonin. *Visual Neuroscience*, 19, 593-601.

Dubocovich, M. L. (1983). Melatonin is a potent modulator of dopamine release in the retina. *Nature* (London), 306, 782-784.

El-Remessy, A. B., Khalil, I. E., Matragoon S, Abou-Mohamed, G., Tsai, N. J., Roon, P., Caldwell, R. B., Caldwell, R. W., Green, K. and Liou, G. I. (2003) Neuroprotective effect of (-) Delta9-tetrahydrocannabinol and cannabidiol in N-methyl-D-aspartate-induced retinal neurotoxicity: involvement of peroxynitrite. *The American Journal of Pathology*, 163,1997-2008.

Faillace MP, Sarmiento MI, Siri LN, Rosenstein RE. (1994). Diurnal variations in cyclic AMP and melatonin content of golden hamster retina. *J. Neurochem.*; 62(5):1995-2000.

Faillace, M. P., Cutrera, R., Sarmiento, M. I. and Rosenstein, R. E. (1995). Evidence for local synthesis of melatonin in golden hamster retina. *Neuroreport*, 6, 2093-2095.

Ferrari, E., Arcaini, A., Gornati, R., Pelanconi, L., Cravello, L., Fioravanti, M., Solerte, S. B. and Magri, F. (2000). Pineal and pituitary-adrenocortical function in physiological aging and in senile dementia. *Experimental Gerontology*, 35, 1239-1250.

Fujieda, H., Hamadanizadeh, S. A., Wankiewicz, E., Pang, S. F. and Brown, G. M. (1999). Expression of mt1 melatonin receptor in rat retina: evidence for multiple cell targets for melatonin. *Neuroscience*, 93, 793-799.

Fujieda, H., Scher, J., Hamadanizadeh, S. A., Wankiewicz, E., Pang, S. F. and Brown, G. M. (2000). Dopaminergic and GABAergic amacrine cells are direct targets of melatonin: immunocytochemical study of mt1 melatonin receptor in guinea pig retina. *Visual Neuroscience*, 17, 63-70.

Fukuhara, C., Dirden, J. C. and Tosini, G. (2001). Photic regulation of melatonin in rat retina and the role of proteasomal proteolysis. *Neuroreport,* 12, 3833-3837.

Fukuhara, C., Liu, C., Ivanova, T. N., Chan, G. C., Storm, D. R., Iuvone, P. M. and Tosini, G. (2004). Gating of the cAMP signaling cascade and melatonin synthesis by the circadian clock in mammalian retina. *Journal of Neuroscience*, 24, 1803-1811.

Gadea, A. and López-Colome, A.M. (2001). Glial transporters for glutamate, glycine, and GABA. II. GABA transporters. *Journal of Neuroscience Research*, 63, 461-468.

Gan, J., Alonso-Gomez, A. L., Avendano, G., Johnson, B. and Iuvone, P. M. (1995). Melatonin biosynthesis in photoreceptor-enriched chick retinal cell cultures: role of cyclic AMP in the K(+)-evoked, Ca(2+)-dependent induction of serotonin N-acetyltransferase activity. *Neurochemistry International*, 27, 147-155.

Garbarino-Pico, E., Carpentieri, A. R., Contin, M. A., Sarmiento, M. I., Brocco, M. A., Panzetta, P., Rosenstein, R. E., Caputto, B. L. and Guido, M. E. (2004). Retinal ganglion cells are autonomous circadian oscillators synthesizing N-acetylserotonin during the day. *The Journal of Biological Chemistry*, 279, 51172-51181.

Gegelashvili, G. and Schousboe, A. (1998). Cellular distribution and kinetic properties of high-affinity glutamate transporters. *Brain Research Bulletin*, 45, 233–238.

Giardino, I., Fard, A.K., Hatchell, D.L. and Brownlee, M. (1998). Aminoguanidine inhibits reactive oxygen species formation, lipid peroxidation, and oxidant-induced apoptosis. *Diabetes* 47, 1114-1120.

Gorovits, R., Avidan, N., Avisar, N., Shaked, I. and Vardimon, L. (1997). Glutamine synthetase protects against neuronal degeneration in injured retinal tissue. *Proceedings of the National Academy of Sciences of the United States of America*, 94, 7024-7029.

Greve, P., Alonso-Gómez, A., Bernard, M., Ma, M., Haque, R., Klein, D. C. and Iuvone, P. M. (1999). Serotonin N-acetyltransferase mRNA levels in photoreceptor-enriched chicken retinal cell cultures: elevation by cyclic AMP. *Journal of Neurochemistry*, 73, 1894-1900.

Grima, G., Cuenod, M., Pfeiffer, S., Mayer, B. and Do, K. Q. (1998). Arginine availability controls the N-methyl-D-aspartate-induced nitric oxide synthesis: involvement of a glial-neuronal arginine transfer. *Journal of Neurochemistry*,71, 2139-2144.

Guenther, A. L., Schmidt, S. I., Laatsch, H., Fotso, S., Ness, H., Ressmeyer, A. R., Poeggeler, B. and Hardeland, R. (2005). Reactions of the melatonin metabolite AMK (N1-acetyl-5-methoxykynuramine) with reactive nitrogen species: formation of novel compounds, 3-acetamidomethyl-6-methoxycinnolinone and 3-nitro-AMK. *Journal of Pineal Research*, 39, 251-260.

Guido, M.E., Garbarino-Pico, E., Contin, M. A., Valdez, D. J., Nieto, P. S., Verra, D. M., Acosta-Rodriguez, V. A., de Zavalía, N. and Rosenstein, R. E. (2010). Inner retinal circadian clocks and non-visual photoreceptors: novel players in the circadian system. *Progress in Neurobiology*, 92, 484-504.

Hall, E. D. (1985). High-dose glucocorticoid treatment improves neurological recovery in head-injured mice. *Journal of Neurosurgery*, 62, 882-887.

Haque, R., Chaurasia, S. S., Wessel, J. H., III and Iuvone, P. M. (2002). Dual regulation of cryptochrome 1 mRNA expression in chicken retina by light and circadian oscillators. *Neuroreport*, 13, 2247-2251.

Hardeland, R. (2005). Antioxidative protection by melatonin: multiplicity of mechanisms from radical detoxification to radical avoidance. *Endocrine*, 27, 119-130.

Hardeland, R., Balzer, I., Poeggeler, B., Fuhrberg, B., Uria, H., Behrmann, G., Wolf, R., Meyer, T. J. and Reiter, R. J. (1995). On the primary functions of melatonin in evolution: mediation of photoperiodic signals in a unicell, photooxidation, and scavenging of free radicals. *Journal of Pineal Research*, 18, 104-111.

Heidinger, V., Hicks, D., Sahel, J. and Dreyfus, H. (1999). Ability of retinal Muller glial cells to protect neurons against excitotoxicity in vitro depends upon maturation and neuron-glial interactions. *Glia*, 25, 229-239.

Holmgren, A. (1989). Thioredoxin and glutaredoxin systems. T*he Journal of Biological Chemistry*, 264, 13963-13966.

Honda, S., Yamamoto, M. and Saito, N. (1995). Immunocytochemical localization of three subtypes of GABA transporter in rat retina. Brain Research. *Molecular Brain Research*, 33, 319-325.

Honkanen, R. A., Baruah, S., Zimmerman, M. B., Khanna, C. L., Weaver, Y. K, Narkiewicz, J., Waziri, R., Gehrs, K. M., Weingeist, T. A., Boldt, H. C., Folk, J. C., Russell, S. R. and Kwon, Y. H. (2003). Vitreous amino acid concentrations in patients with glaucoma undergoing vitrectomy. *Archives of Ophthalmology*, 121, 183-188.

Ianas, O., Olinescu, R. and Badescu, I. (1991). Melatonin involvement in oxidative processes. *Endocrinologie*, 29, 147-153.

Imbesi, M., Uz, T. and Manev, H. (2008). Role of melatonin receptors in the effects of melatonin on BDNF and neuroprotection in mouse cerebellar neurons. *Journal of Neural Transmission*, 115, 1495-1499.

Itoh, M. T., Takahashi, N., Abe, M. and Shimizu, K. (2007). Expression and cellular localization of melatonin-synthesizing enzymes in the rat lens. *Journal of Pineal Research*, 42, 92-96.

Iuvone, P. M., Brown, A. D., Haque, R., Weller, J., Zawilska, J. B., Chaurasia, S. S., Ma, M. and Klein, D. C. (2002). Retinal melatonin production: role of proteasomal proteolysis in circadian and photic control of arylalkylamine N-acetyltransferase. *Investigative Ophthalmology and Visual Science*, 43, 564-572.

Ivanova, T. N. and Iuvone, P. M. (2003). Melatonin synthesis in retina: circadian regulation of arylalkylamine N-acetyltransferase activity in cultured photoreceptor cells of embryonic chicken retina. *Brain Research*, 973, 56-63.

Jimenez-Jorge, S., Guerrero, J. M., Jimenez-Caliani, J., Naranjo, M. C., Lardone, P. J., Carrillo-Vico, A., Osuna, C. and Molinero, P. (2007). Evidence for melatonin synthesis in the rat brain during development. *Journal of Pineal Research*, 42, 240-246.

Johnson, J., Chen, T. K., Rickman, D. W., Evans, C. and Brecha, N. C. (1996). Multiple gamma-Aminobutyric acid plasma membrane transporters (GAT-1, GAT-2, GAT-3) in the rat retina. *The Journal of Comparative Neurology*, 375, 212-224.

Kalloniatis, M. and Tomisich, G. (1999). Amino acid neurochemistry of the vertebrate retina. *Progress in Retinal and Eye Research*, 18, 811-866.

Kawasaki, A., Otori, Y. and Barnstable, C. J. (2000). Müller cell protection of rat retinal ganglion cells from glutamate and nitric oxide neurotoxicity. *Investigative Ophthalmology and Visual Science*, 41, 3444-3450.

Kong, X., Li, X., Cai, Z., Yang, N., Liu, Y., Shu, J., Pan, L. and Zuo, P. (2008). Melatonin regulates the viability and differentiation of rat midbrain neural stem cells. *Cellular and Molecular Neurobiology*, 28,569-579.

Kortuem, K., Geiger, L. K. and Levin, L. A. (2000). Differential susceptibility of retinal ganglion cells to reactive oxygen species. *Investigative Ophthalmology and Visual Science*, 41, 3176-3182.

Kurysheva, N. I., Vinetskaia, M. I., Erichev, V. P., Demchuk, M. L. and Kuryshev, S. I. (1996). Contribution of free-radical reactions of chamber humor to the development of primary open-angle glaucoma. *Vestnik Oftalmologii*, 112, 3-5.

Kurz, S. and Harrison, D. (1997). Insulin and the arginine paradox. *The Journal of Clinical Investigation*, 99, 369-370.

León, J., Vives, F., Crespo, E., Camacho, E., Espinosa, A., Gallo, M. A., Escames, G. and Acuña-Castroviejo, D. (1998). Modification of nitric oxide synthase activity and neuronal response in rat striatum by melatonin and kynurenine derivatives. *Journal of Neuroendocrinology*, 10, 297-302.

León, J., Acuña-Castroviejo, D., Sainz, R. M., Mayo, J. C., Tan, D. X. and Reiter, R. J. (2004). Melatonin and mitochondrial function. *Life Sciences*, 75, 765-790.

León, J., Acuña-Castroviejo, D., Escames, G., Tan, D. X. and Reiter, R. J. (2005). Melatonin mitigates mitochondrial malfunction. *Journal of Pineal Research*, 38, 1-9.

Levkovitch-Verbin, H., Martin, K. R., Quigley, H. A., Baumrind, L. A., Pease, M. E. and Valenta, D. (2002). Measurement of amino acid levels in the vitreous humor of rats after chronic intraocular pressure elevation or optic nerve transection. *Journal of Glaucoma*, 11, 396-405.

Liu, B. and Neufeld, A. H. (2000). Expression of nitric oxide synthase-2 (NOS-2) in reactive astrocytes of the human glaucomatous optic nerve head. *Glia.*, 30, 178-186.

Liu, B. and Neufeld, A. H. (2001). Nitric oxide synthase-2 in human optic nerve head astrocytes induced by elevated pressure in vitro. *Archives of Ophthalmology*, 119, 240-245.

Liu, B. and Neufeld, A. H. (2003). Activation of epidermal growth factor receptor signals induction of nitric oxide synthase-2 in human optic nerve head astrocytes in glaucomatous optic neuropathy. *Neurobiology of Disease*, 13, 109-123.

Liu, C., Fukuhara, C., Wessel, J. H., III, Iuvone, P. M. and Tosini, G. (2004). Localization of Aa-nat mRNA in the rat retina by fluorescence in situ hybridization and laser capture microdissection. *Cell and Tissue Research*, 315, 197-201.

Liu, F., Yuan, H., Sugamori, K. S., Hamadanizadeh, A., Lee, F. J., Pang, S. F., Brown, G. M., Pristupa, Z. B. and Niznik, H. B. (1995). Molecular and functional characterization of a partial cDNA encoding a novel chicken brain melatonin receptor. *FEBS Letters*, 374, 273-278.

Liversidge, J., Dick, A. and Gordon, S. (2002). Nitric oxide mediates apoptosis through formation of peroxynitrite and Fas/Fas-ligand interactions in experimental autoimmune uveitis. *The American Journal of Pathology*, 160, 905-916.

Long, D. J., Iskander, K., Gaikwad, A., Arin, M., Roop, D. R., Knox, R., Barrios, R. and Jaiswal, A. K. (2002). Disruption of dihydronicotinamide riboside:quinone oxidoreductase 2 (NQO2) leads to myeloid hyperplasia of bone marrow and decreased sensitivity to menadione toxicity. *The Journal of Biological Chemistry*, 277, 46131-46139.

López-Costa, J. J., Goldstein, J., Pecci-Saavedra, J., Della Maggiore, V. M., De Las Heras, M. A., Sarmiento, M. I. and Rosenstein, R. E. (1999). GABA release mechanism in the golden hamster retina. *The International Journal of Neuroscience*, 98, 13-25.

Louzada-Junior, P., Dias, J. J., Santos, W. F., Lachat, J. J., Bradford, H. F. and Coutinho-Netto, J. (1992). Glutamate release in experimental ischaemia of the retina: an approach using microdialysis. *Journal of Neurochemistry*, 59, 358-363.

Lundmark, P. O., Pandi-Perumal, S. R., Srinivasan, V. and Cardinali, D. P. (2006). Role of melatonin in the eye and ocular dysfunctions. *Visual Neuroscience*, 23, 853-862.

Lundmark, P. O., Pandi-Perumal, S. R., Srinivasan, V., Cardinali, D. P. and Rosenstein, R. E. (2007). Melatonin in the eye: implications for glaucoma. *Experimental Eye Research*, 84, 1021-1030.

Manabe, S., Gu, Z. and Lipton, S. A. (2005). Activation of matrix metalloproteinase-9 via neuronal nitric oxide synthase contributes to NMDA-induced retinal ganglion cell death. *Investigative Ophthalmology and Visual Science*, 46, 4747-4753.

Marchiafava, P. L. and Longoni, B. (1999). Melatonin as an antioxidant in retinal photoreceptors. *Journal of Pineal Research*, 26, 184-189.

Marcic, T. S., Belyea, D. A. and Katz, B. (2003). Neuroprotection in glaucoma: a model for neuroprotection in optic neuropathies. *Current Opinion in Ophthalmology*, 14, 353-356.

Martin, X. D., Malina, H. Z., Brennan, M. C., Hendrickson, P. H. and Lichter, P. R. (1992). The ciliary body--the third organ found to synthesize indoleamines in humans. *European Journal of Ophthalmology*, 2, 67-72.

Martin, K. R., Levkovitch-Verbin, H., Valenta, D., Baumrind, L., Pease, M. E. and Quigley, H. A. (2002). Retinal glutamate transporter changes in experimental glaucoma and after optic nerve transection in the rat. *Investigative Ophthalmology and Visual Science*, 43, 2236-2243.

Martinez-Ruiz, A. and Lamas, S. (2004). S-nitrosylation: a potential new paradigm in signal transduction. *Cardiovascular Research.*, 62, 43-52.

Melino, G., Bernassola, F., Knight, R. A., Corasaniti, M. T., Nistico, G. and Finazzi-Agro, A. (1997). S-nitrosylation regulates apoptosis. *Nature*, 388, 432-433.

Meyer, P., Pache, M., Loeffler, K. U., Brydon, L., Jockers, R., Flammer, J., Wirz-Justice, A. and Savaskan, E. (2002). Melatonin MT-1-receptor immunoreactivity in the human eye. *British Journal of. Ophthalmology*, 86, 1053-1057.

Mhatre, M. C., van Jaarsveld, A. S. and Reiter, R. J. (1988). Melatonin in the lacrimal gland: first demonstration and experimental manipulation. *Biochemical and Biophysical Research Communications*, 153, 1186-1192.

Moreno, M. C., Campanelli, J., Sande, P., Sanez, D. A., Keller Sarmiento, M. I. and Rosenstein, R. E. (2004). Retinal oxidative stress induced by high intraocular pressure. *Free Radical Biology and Medicine*, 37, 803-812.

Moreno, M. C., Sande, P., Marcos, H. A., de Zavalía, N., Keller Sarmiento, M. I. and Rosenstein, R.E. (2005a). Effect of glaucoma on the retinal glutamate/glutamine cycle activity. *The FASEB Journal*, 19, 1161-1162.

Moreno, M. C., Marcos, H. J., Croxatto, J. O., Sande, P. H., Campanelli, J., Jaliffa, C. O., Benozzi, J. and Rosenstein, R. E. (2005b) A new experimental model of glaucoma in rats through intracameral injections of hyaluronic acid. *Experimental Eye Research*, 81, 71-80.

Moreno, M. C., de Zavalía, N., Sande, P., Jaliffa, C. O., Fernandez, D. C., Keller Sarmiento, M. I. and Rosenstein, R. E. (2008). Effect of ocular hypertension on retinal GABAergic activity. *Neurochemistry International*, 52, 675-82.

Morrison, J. C., Moore, C. G., Deppmeier, L. M., Gold, B.G., Meshul, C.K. and Johnson, E. C. (1997). A rat model of chronic pressure-induced optic nerve damage. *Experimental Eye Research*, 64, 85-96.

Mosinger, J. L., Price, M. T., Bai, H. Y., Xiao, H., Wozniak, D. F. and Olney, J. W. (1991). Blockade of both NMDA and non-NMDA receptors is required for optimal protection against ischemic neuronal degeneration in the in vivo adult mammalian retina. *Experimental Neurology.*, 113, 10-17.

Namihira, M., Honma, S., Abe, H., Masubuchi, S., Ikeda, M. and Honmaca, K. (2001). Circadian pattern, light responsiveness and localization of rPer1 and rPer2 gene expression in the rat retina. *Neuroreport*, 12, 471-475.

Naskar, R., Vorwerk, C. K. and Dreyer, E. B. (2000). Concurrent downregulation of a glutamate transporter and receptor in glaucoma. *Investigative Ophthalmology and Visual Science*, 41, 1940-1944.

Neufeld, A. H. (2004). Pharmacologic neuroprotection with an inhibitor of nitric oxide synthase for the treatment of glaucoma. *Brain Research Bulletin.*, 62, 455-459.

Neufeld, A. H., Hernandez, M. R. and Gonzalez, M. (1997). Nitric oxide synthase in the human glaucomatous optic nerve head. *Archives of Ophthalmology*, 115, 497-503.

Neufeld, A. H., Sawada, A. and Becker, B. (1999). Inhibition of nitric-oxide synthase 2 by aminoguanidine provides neuroprotection of retinal ganglion cells in a rat model of chronic glaucoma. *Proceedings of the National Academy of Sciences of the United States of America*, 96, 9944-9948.

Niki, T., Hamada, T., Ohtomi, M., Sakamoto, K., Suzuki, S., Kako, K., Hosoya, Y., Horikawa, K. and Ishida, N. (1998). The localization of the site of arylalkylamine N-acetyltransferase circadian expression in the photoreceptor cells of mammalian retina. *Biochemical and Biophysical Research Communications*, 248, 115-120.

Niles, L. P., Armstrong, K. J., Castro, L. M. R., Dao, C. V., Sharma, R., McMillan, C. R., Doering, L. C. and Kirkham, D. L. (2004). Neural stem cells express melatonin receptors and neurotrophic factors: colocalization of the MT1 receptor with neuronal and glial markers. *BMC Neuroscience*, 5, 41.

Nosjean, O., Ferro, M., Coge, F., Beauverger, P., Henlin, J. M., Lefoulon, F., Fauchere, J. L., Delagrange, P., Canet, E. and Boutin, J. A. (2000). Identification of the melatonin-binding site MT3 as the quinone reductase 2. *The Journal of Biological Chemistry*, 275, 31311-31317.

Nucci, C., Tartaglione, R., Rombola, L., Morrone, L.A., Fazzi, E. and Bagetta, G., (2005). Neurochemical evidence to implicate elevated glutamate in the mechanisms of high intraocular pressure (IOP)-induced retinal ganglion cell death in rat. *Neurotoxicology,* 26, 935-941.

Ohta, Y., Yamasaki, T., Niwa, T., Niimi, K., Majima, Y. and Ishiguro, I. (1996). Role of catalase in retinal antioxidant defence system: its comparative study among rabbits, guinea pigs, and rats. *Ophthalmic Research.*, 28, 336-342.

Osborne, N.. N., Nash, M. S. and Wood, J. P. (1998). Melatonin counteracts ischemia-induced apoptosis in human retinal pigment epithelial cells. *Investigative Ophthalmology and Visual Science*, 39, 2374-2383.

Osborne, N. N., Chidlow, G., Nash, M. S. and Wood, J. P. (1999). The potential of neuroprotection in glaucoma treatment. *Current Opinion in Ophthalmology*, 10, 82-92.

Otis, T. S. and Jahr, C. E. (1998). Anion currents and predicted glutamate flux through a neuronal glutamate transporter. *The Journal of Neuroscience*, 18, 7099-7110.

Pandi-Perumal, S. R., Srinivasan, V., Maestroni, G. J., Cardinali, D. P., Poeggeler, B. and Hardeland, R. (2006). Melatonin: Nature's most versatile biological signal? *The FEBS Journal*, 273, 2813-2838.

Pang, I. .H., Johnson, E. C., Jia, L., Cepurna, W. O., Shepard, A. R., Hellberg, M. R., Clark, A. F. and Morrison, J. C. (2005). Evaluation of inducible nitric oxide synthase in glaucomatous optic neuropathy and pressureinduced optic nerve damage. *Investigative Ophthalmology and Visual Science*, 6, 1313-1321.

Patel, A. J., Hunt, A. and Tahourdin, C. S. (1983). Regulation of in vivo glutamine synthetase activity by glucocorticoids in the developing rat brain. *Brain Research*, 312, 83-91.

Pierce, M. E. and Besharse, J. C. (1985). Circadian regulation of retinomotor movements. I. Interaction of melatonin and dopamine in the control of cone length. *Journal of General Physiology*, 86, 671-689.

Poitry, S., Poitry-Yamate, C., Ueberfeld, J., MacLeish, P. R. and Tsacopoulos, M. (2000). Mechanisms of glutamate metabolic signaling in retinal glial (Müller) cells. *The Journal of Neuroscience*, 20, 1809-1821.

Pow, D. V. and Robinson, S. R. (1994). Glutamate in some retinal neurons is derived solely from glia. *Neuroscience*, 60, 355-366.

Pozo, D., Reiter, R. J., Calvo, J. R. and Guerrero, J. M. (1997). Inhibition of cerebellar nitric oxide synthase and cyclic GMP production by melatonin via complex formation with calmodulin. *Journal of Cellular Biochemistry*, 65, 430-442.

Rada, J. A. and Wiechmann, A. F. (2006). Melatonin receptors in chick ocular tissues: implications for a role of melatonin in ocular growth regulation. *Investigative Ophthalmology and Visual Science*, 47, 25-33.

Rajesh, M., Sulochana, K. N., Punitham, R., Biswas, J., Lakshmi, S. and Ramakrishnan, S. (2003). Involvement of oxidative and nitrosative stress in promoting retinal vasculitis in patients with Eales' disease. *Clinical Biochemistry*, 36, 377-385.

Reiter, R. J., Tan, D. X., Poeggeler, B., Menendez-Pelaez, A., Chen, L. D. and Saarela, S. (1994). Melatonin as a free radical scavenger: implications for aging and age-related diseases. *Annals of the New York Academy of Sciences*, 719, 1-12.

Reiter, R. J., Guerrero, J. M., Escames, G., Pappolla, M. A. and Acuña-Castroviejo, D. (1997). Prophylactic actions of melatonin in oxidative neurotoxicity. Annals *of the New York Academy of Sciences*, 825, 70-78.

Reiter, R. J., Garcia, J. J. and Pie, J. (1998). Oxidative toxicity in models of neurodegeneration: responses to melatonin. *Restorative Neurology and Neuroscience*, 12, 135-142.

Reiter, R. J., Cabrera, J., Sainz, R. M., Mayo, J. C., Manchester, L. C. and Tan, D. X. (1999). Melatonin as a pharmacological agent against neuronal loss in experimental models of Huntington's disease, Alzheimer's disease and parkinsonism. *Annals of the New York Academy of Sciences*, 890, 471-485.

Reiter, R. J., Tan, D. X., Osuna, C. and Gitto, E. (2000). Actions of melatonin in the reduction of oxidative stress. A review. *Journal of Biomedical Science*, 7, 444-458.

Reiter, R. J., Tan, D. X., Manchester, L. C., Simopoulos, A. P., Maldonado, M. D., Flores, L. J. and Terron, M. P. (2007). Melatonin in edible plants (phytomelatonin): Identification, concentrations, bioavailability and proposed functions. *World Review of Nutrition and Dietetics*, 97, 211-230.

Reppert, S. M., Godson, C., Mahle, C. D., Weaver, D. R., Slaugenhaupt, S. A. and Gusella, J. F. (1995). Molecular characterization of a second melatonin receptor expressed in human retina and brain: the Mel1b melatonin receptor. *Proceedings of the National Academy of Sciences of the United States of America*, 92, 8734-8738.

Riepe, R. E. and Norenburg, M. D. (1977). Muller cell localization of glutamine synthetase in rat retina. *Nature,* 268, 654-655.

Rosenstein, R. E. and Cardinali, D. P. (1986). Melatonin increases in vivo GABA accumulation in rat hypothalamus, cerebellum, cerebral cortex and pineal gland. *Brain Research*, 98, 403-406.

Rosenstein, R. E., Estévez, A. G. and Cardinali, D. P. (1989). Time-dependent effect of melatonin on glutamic acid decarboxylase activity and Cl influx in rat hypothalamus. *Journal of Neuroendocrinology*, 1, 443-447.

Rosner, M., Lam, T. T. and Tso, M. O. (1992). Therapeutic parameters of methylprednisolone treatment for retinal photic injury in a rat model. *Research Communications in Chemical Pathology and Pharmacology*, 77, 299-311.

Rufiange, M., Dumont, M. and Lachapelle, P. (2002). Correlating retinal function with melatonin secretion in subjects with an early or late circadian phase. *Investigative Ophthalmology and Visual Science*, 43, 2491-2499.

Sáenz, D. A, Cymeryng, C. B., De Nichilo, A., Sacca, G. .B., Keller Sarmiento, M.. I. and Rosenstein, R. E. (2002a). Photic regulation of L-arginine uptake in the golden hamster retina. *Journal of Neurochemistry*, 80, 512-519.

Sáenz, D.A., Turjanski, A. G., Sacca, G. B., Marti, M., Doctorovich, F., Sarmiento, M. I., Estrin, D. A. and Rosenstein, R. E. (2002b). Physiological concentrations of melatonin inhibit the nitridergic pathway in the Syrian hamster retina. *Journal of Pineal Research*, 33, 31-36.

Sáenz, D. A., Goldin, A. P., Minces, L., Chianelli, M., Sarmiento, M. I. and Rosenstein R. E. (2004). Effect of melatonin on the retinal glutamate/glutamine cycle in the golden hamster retina. *The FASEB Journal*, 18,1912-3.

Samples, J. R., Krause, G. and Lewy, A. J. (1988). Effect of melatonin on intraocular pressure. *Current Eye Research*, 7, 649-653.

Sande, P. H., Fernandez, D. C., Aldana Marcos, H. J., Chianelli, M. S., Aisemberg, J., Silberman, D. M., Sáenz, D. A. and Rosenstein, R. E. (2008). Therapeutic effect of melatonin in experimental uveitis. *The American Journal of Pathology*, 173, 1702-1713.

Sarkar, P. K. and Chaudhury, S. (1983). Messenger RNA for glutamine synthetase. *Molecular and Cellular Biochemistry*, 53-54, 233-244.

Sarthy, P. V. and Lam, D. M. (1978). Biochemical studies of isolated glial (Müller) cells from the turtle retina. *The Journal of Cell Biology*, 78, 675-684.

Savaskan, E., Wirz-Justice, A., Olivieri, G., Pache, M., Krauchi, K., Brydon, L., Jockers, R., Muller-Spahn, F. and Meyer, P. (2002). Distribution of melatonin MT1 receptor immunoreactivity in human retina. *The Journal of Histochemistry and Cytochemistry*, 50, 519-526.

Savaskan, E., Jockers, R., Ayoub, M., Angeloni, D., Fraschini, F., Flammer, J., Eckert, A., Muller-Spahn, F. and Meyer, P. (2007). The MT2 melatonin receptor subtype is present in human retina and decreases in Alzheimer's disease. *Current Alzheimer Research*, 4, 47-51.

Scher, J., Wankiewicz, E., Brown, G. M. and Fujieda, H. (2002). MT(1) melatonin receptor in the human retina: expression and localization. *Investigative Ophthalmology and Visual Science*, 43, 889-897.

Scher, J., Wankiewicz, E., Brown, G. M. and Fujieda, H. (2003). AII amacrine cells express the MT1 melatonin receptor in human and macaque retina. *Experimental Eye Research*, 77, 375-382.

Schwartz, E. A. (1987). Depolarization without calcium can release gammaaminobutyric acid from a retinal neuron. *Science*, 238, 350-355.

Sen, C. K. (1998). Redox signaling and the emerging therapeutic potential of thiol antioxidants. *Biochemical Pharmacology*, 55, 1747-1758.

Shareef, S. R., Garcia-Valenzuela, E., Salierno, A., Walsh, J. and Sharma, S.C. (1995). Chronic ocular hypertension following episcleral venous occlusion in rats. *Experimental Eye Research*, 61, 379-382.

Shen, F., Chen, B., Danias, J., Lee, K. C., Lee, H., Su, Y., Podos, S. M. and Mittag, T. W. J. (2004). Glutamate-induced glutamine synthetase expression in retinal Muller cells after shortterm ocular hypertension in the rat. *Investigative Ophthalmology and Visual Science*, 45, 3107-3112.

Simonian, N. A. and Coyle, J. T. (1996). Oxidative stress in neurodegenerative diseases. *Annual Review of Pharmacology and Toxicology*, 36, 83-106.

Siu, A. W., Reiter, R. J. and To, C. H. (1999). Pineal indoleamines and vitamin E reduce nitric oxide-induced lipid peroxidation in rat retinal homogenates. *Journal of Pineal Research*, 27, 122-128.

Siu, A. W., Maldonado, M., Sanchez-Hidalgo, M., Tan, D. X. and Reiter, R. J. (2006). Protective effects of melatonin in experimental free radical-related ocular diseases. *Journal of Pineal Research*, 40, 101-109.

Spector, A., Yang, Y., Ho, Y. S., Magnenat, J. L., Wang, R. R., Ma, W. and Li, W. C. (1996).Variation in cellular glutathione peroxidase activity in lens epithelial cells, transgenics and knockouts does not significantly change the response to H2O2 stress. *Experimental Eye Research*, 62, 521-540;

Srinivasan, V., Pandi-Perumal, S. R., Maestroni, G. J., Esquifino, A. I., Hardeland, R. and Cardinali, D. P. (2005). Role of melatonin in neurodegenerative diseases. *Neurotoxicity Research*, 7, 293-318.

Srinivasan, V., Pandi-Perumal, S. R., Cardinali, D. P., Poeggeler, B. and Hardeland, R. (2006). Melatonin in Alzheimer's disease and other neurodegenerative disorders. *Behavioral and Brain Functions*, 2, 15.

Stevens, B. R., Kakuda, D. K., Yu, K., Waters, M., Vo, C.B. and Raizada, M. K. (1996). Induced nitric oxide synthesis is dependent on induced alternatively spliced CAT-2 encoding L-arginine transport in brain astrocytes. *The Journal of Biological Chemistry*, 271, 24017-24022.

Tan, D. X., Manchester, L. C., Terron, M. P., Flores, L. J. and Reiter, R. J. (2007a). One molecule, many derivatives: a never-ending interaction of melatonin with reactive oxygen and nitrogen species? *Journal of Pineal Research*, 42, 28-42.

Tan, D. X., Manchester, L. C., Terron, M. P., Flores, L. J., Tamura, H. and Reiter, R. J. (2007b). Melatonin as a naturally occurring co-substrate of quinone reductase-2, the putative MT3 melatonin membrane receptor: hypothesis and significance. *Journal of Pineal Research*, 43, 317-320.

Tanaka, K. (2000). Functions of glutamate transporters in the brain. *Neuroscience Research*, 37, 15-19.

Tang, Q., Hu, Y. and Cao, Y. (2006). Neuroprotective effect of melatonin on retinal ganglion cells in rats. Journal of Huazhong University of Science and Technology. *Medical Sciences*, 26, 235-237, 253.

Tanito, M., Nishiyama, A., Tanaka, T., Masutani, H., Nakamura, H., Yodoi, J. and Ohira, A. (2002). Change of redox status and modulation by thiol replenishment in retinal photooxidative damage. *Investigative Ophthalmology and Visual Science*, 43, 2392-2400.

Tezel, G. (2006). Oxidative stress in glaucomatous neurodegeneration: mechanisms and consequences. *Progress in Retinal and Eye Research*, 25, 490-513.

Thompson, C. L., Selby, C. P., Partch, C. L., Plante, D. T., Thresher, R. J., Araujo, F. and Sancar, A. (2004). Further evidence for the role of cryptochromes in retinohypothalamic photoreception/phototransduction. Brain Research. *Molecular Brain Research*, 122, 158-166.

Thoreson, W. B. and Witkovsky, P. (1999). Glutamate receptors and circuits in the vertebrate retina. *Progress in Retinal and Eye Research*, 18, 765-810.

Tosini, G. (2000). Melatonin circadian rhythm in the retina of mammals. *Chronobiology International,* 17, 599-612.

Tosini, G. and Menaker, M. (1996). Circadian rhythms in cultured mammalian retina. *Science*, 272, 419-421.

Tosini, G. and Menaker, M. (1998). The clock in the mouse retina: melatonin synthesis and photoreceptor degeneration. *Brain Research*, 789, 221-228.

Tosini, G., Chaurasia, S. S. and Michael, I. P. (2006). Regulation of arylalkylamine N-acetyltransferase (AANAT) in the retina. *Chronobiology International*, 23, 381-391.

Tosini, G., Pozdeyev, N., Sakamoto, K. and Iuvone, P. M. (2008). The circadian clock system in the mammalian retina. *Bioessays*, 30, 624-633.

Turjanski, A. G., Rosenstein, R. E. and Estrin, D. A. (1998). Reactions of melatonin and related indoles with free radicals: a computational study. *Journal of Medicinal Chemistry*, 41, 3684-3689.

Turjanski, A. G., Leonik, F., Rosenstein, R. E. and Doctorovich, F. (2000). Scavenging of NO by melatonin. *Journal of the American Chemical Society*, 122, 10468-10469.

Ueda, J., Sawaguchi, S., Hanyu, T., Yaoeda, K., Fukuchi, T., Abe, H. and Ozawa, H. (1998). Experimental glaucoma model in the rat induced by laser trabecular photocoagulation after an intracameral injection of India ink. *Japanese Journal of Ophthalmology*. 42, 337-344.

van Reyk, D. M., Gillies, M. C. and Davies, M. J. (2003). The retina: oxidative stress and diabetes. *Redox Report.*, 8, 187-192.

Verkerk, A. and Jongkind, J. F. (1992). Vascular cells under peroxide induced oxidative stress: a balance study on in vitro peroxide handling by vascular endothelial and smooth muscle cells. *Free Radical Research Communications*, 17, 121-132.

Vorwerk, C. K., Hyman, B. T., Miller, J. W., Husain, D., Zurakowski, D., Huang, P. L., Fishman, M. C. and Dreyer, E. B. (1997). The role of neuronal and endothelial nitric oxide synthase in retinal excitotoxicity. *Investigative Ophthalmology and Visual Science*, 38, 2038-2044.

Vorwerk, C. K., Naskar, R., Schuettauf, F., Quinto, K., Zurakowski, D., Gochenauer, G., Robinson, M. B., Mackler, S. A. and Dreyer, E. B. (2000). Depression of retinal glutamate transporter function leads to elevated intravitreal glutamate levels and ganglion cell death. *Investigative Ophthalmology and Visual Science*, 41, 3615-3621.

Wamsley, S., Gabelt, B. T., Dahl, D. B., Case, G. L., Sherwood, R. W., May, C. A., Hernandez, M. R. and Kaufman, P. L. (2005). Vitreous glutamate concentration and axon loss in monkeys with experimental glaucoma. *Archives of Ophthalmology*, 123, 64-70.

Weber, A. J., Harman, C. D. and Viswanathan, S. (2008). Effects of optic nerve injury, glaucoma, and neuroprotection on the survival, structure, and function of ganglion cells in the mammalian retina. *The Journal of Physiology*, 586, 4393-4400.

White, M. P. and Fisher, L. J. (1989). Effects of exogenous melatonin on circadian disc shedding in the albino rat retina. *Vision Research*, 29, 167-179.

Wiechmann, A. F. and Rada, J. A. (2003). Melatonin receptor expression in the cornea and sclera. *Experimental Eye Research*, 77, 219-225.

Wiechmann, A. F. and Summers, J. A. (2008). Circadian rhythms in the eye: the physiological significance of melatonin receptors in ocular tissues. *Progress in Retinal and Eye Research*, 27, 137-160.

Wiechmann, A. F. and Wirsig-Wiechmann, C. R. (2001). Multiple cell targets for melatonin action in Xenopus laevis retina: distribution of melatonin receptor immunoreactivity. *Visual Neuroscience*, 18, 695-702.

Wiechmann, A. F., Udin, S. B. and Summers Rada, J. A. (2004). Localization of Mel1b melatonin receptor-like immunoreactivity in ocular tissues of Xenopus laevis. *Experimental Eye Research*, 79, 585-594.

Witkovsky, P., Veisenberger, E., Lesauter, J., Yan, L., Johnson, M., Zhang, D. Q., McMahon, D. and Silver, R. (2003). Cellular location and circadian rhythm of expression of the biological clock gene Period 1 in the mouse retina. *The Journal of Neuroscience*, 23, 7670-7676.

Wu, G. S., Zhang, J. and Rao, N. A. (1997). Peroxynitrite and oxidative damage in experimental autoimmune uveitis. *Investigative Ophthalmology and Visual Science*, 38, 1333-1339.

Yang, X. L. (2004). Characterization of receptors for glutamate and GABA in retinal neurons. *Progress in Neurobiology*, 73, 127-150.

In: Glaucoma: Etiology, Pathogenesis and Treatments
Editors: Z. G. Fei and S. Zeng

ISBN: 978-1-61470-975-6
© 2012 Nova Science Publishers, Inc.

Chapter III

Ocular Tissue Changes and Glaucoma Treatment

Cristiana Valente and Michele Iester[*]

Laboratorio clinico anatomo-funzionale per la diagnosi e il trattamento del glaucoma e delle malattie neurooftalmologiche, Clinica Oculistica, Department of Neurological Sciences, Ophthalmology, Genetic, University of Genoa, Italy

INTRODUCTION

Primary open angle glaucoma (POAG) is the leading cause of irreversible and preventable visual field loss. Glaucoma is responsible for 14% of blindness worldwide and it is the second cause of blindness after cataract [1]. In the world, the primary glaucoma afflicts about 60-70 million people, of whom 10% are believed to be bilaterally blind [2,3,4]. POAG is characterized by a progressive optic neuropathy and it is usually asymptomatic until advanced. The most important risk factors include elevated intraocular pressure (IOP), positive family history, advanced age and African ancestry. The pathogenesis of glaucoma is not yet totally explained. POAG can occur with or without raised eye pressure, but nowadays an elevated intraocular pressure remains the main target to whom we can address the treatment: drugs, laser or surgery [5,6,7,8]. Glaucoma remains a major public health problem worldwide. Even in developed countries, half of glaucoma cases are undiagnosed until visual field changes arise. When the diagnosis of glaucoma has been made, patients need lifelong sight checking to prevent progression of visual field damage and to maintain a sighted lifetime. Glaucoma is commonly treated with daily eye-drop drugs to avoid the onset of further irreversible optic nerve damage and visual field defects [9].

As a chronic disease, glaucoma require for a long time a topical treatment whose active agents can have some local and systemic side effects. In a multi-dose bottles, usually used for

---

[*] *Corresponding author:* Michele Iester, MD, PhD Clinica Oculistica, Università di Genova Viale Benedetto XV, 5 16132 Genova Telephone: 00 39 010353 8469 – 7783 Fax: 0103538494 e-mail: iester@unige.it

glaucoma therapy, there are preservatives important to avoid contamination by common pathogens but also responsible of ocular toxicity. Several epidemiologic studies have showed that a chronic use of anti-glaucoma drugs could lead to ocular surface changes (tear film, cornea, conjunctiva) causing ocular discomfort [10,11].

In this chapter we analyzed the ocular changes due to the local treatment and to the preservatives, and in particular to benzalkonium chloride (BAK), that is the most common among all the preservatives. From some years, the use of alternative preservatives with a lighter toxicity or antiglaucoma preservative-free drugs are now available on trade. They could be useful to minimize side effects of glaucoma medications on ocular tissues and increase the patient's compliance because of the higher tolerability of this new drugs [12,13].

IOP-LOWERING AGENTS AND THEIR SIDE EFFECTS

Topical medication is mainly used as first-choice therapy and it should start with one drug. Theoretically, if more than two or three medications are required to control the disease, then other types of treatment, such as laser trabeculoplasty or surgery, should be considered. Surgery is reserved in case of intolerance to topical drugs or in presence of disease progression despite a maximal IOP-lowering therapy. Treatment of glaucoma consists of topical or systemic intraocular pressure lowering agents. Six different classes of IOP-lowering molecules are currently available, including alpha adrenergic agonists, beta-blockers, carbonic anhydrase inhibitor (CAI) (topical and systemic), parasympathomimetics, prostaglandin analogues and sympathomimetics. The efficacy of these classes of glaucomatous drugs are different. The prostaglandins/prostamides cause the biggest intra-ocular pressure decrease among all the lowering agents. They increase uveoscleral outflow resulting in reductions of IOP of between 25 and 35%. Alpha adrenergic agonists, pilocarpine and beta-blockers decrease IOP about 20-25% and topical CAI about 18% [14]. Alpha adrenergic agonists work decreasing aqueous humor production and increasing aqueous humor outflow. B-Blockers and topical CAI decrease IOP by reduction of the aqueous humor production, while parasympathomimetics by increase in facility of outflow of aqueous humor [15]. Many antiglaucoma drugs are available, and the choice of therapy must take into account not only the aims of therapy, but also their mode of action, local and systemic side effects of each medication, cost, quality of life and compliance of patients [15].

The purpose of this chapter is to investigate the effects of glaucoma medication on body tissue and in particular on ocular tissue.

β-blockers and α-2-selective agonist are proved to have a lot of systemic side effects in comparison with the prostaglandin and CAI. β-blockers are responsible of bradycardia, arrhythmias, heart failure, syncope, hypotension, bronchospasm, airways obstruction, elevated serum lipids, increased falls in the ederly. Both β-blockers and α-2-selective agonist can cause drowsiness, anergy, fatigue, dry mouth. It is important to remember that brimonidine should be use carefully in infants because it can lead to apnoea.

β-blockers and adrenergic antagonists have more important systemic side effects than ocular ones. The epithelial keratopathy and light reduction in corneal sensitivity can be the ocular side effects of β-blockers, but they are uncommon. α-2-selective adrenergic agonist can lead to lid elevation, periocular contact dermatitis, conjunctival hyperemia and allergic conjunctivitis. Pupil dilatation has been described in patients who use apraclonidine [16].

Among the adrenergic agonists, a non selective adrenergic agonist such as epinephrine can cause follicular conjunctivitis and macular edema in aphakic eye. The systemic side effects of epinephrine can be the onset of tachycardia, arrhythmias and hypertension [16].

The most potent antiglaucoma agents, the prostaglandin analogs and prostamides cause more frequently ocular side effects such as conjunctival hyperemia, changes in pigmentation of iris, that is permanent, and in pigmentation of periocular skin and in length and number of eyelashes that are reversible. Patients using prostaglandin can suffer of stinging, burning, itching and foreign body sensation but cystoids macular edema, both in pseudophakic and aphakic eyes, remains the most dangerous and fortunately rare ocular effects. Patients that suffer from uveitis should also advice of the possibility of reactivation of herpes keratitis and anterior uveitis [16].

Also the topical carbonic anhydrase inhibitors cause mainly ocular side effects for example superficial punctate keratitis, tearing, burning, stinging, bitter taste, blurred vision for transient myopia. While topical CAI can be responsible just of headache, urticaria, angioedema, pruritus, asthenia, mild paresthesia, the systemic effects of systemic carbonic anhydrase inhibitors are most important such as strong paresthesia, hearing disfunction, loss of appetite, taste alteration, nausea, vomiting, diarrhea, depression, decrease libido, kidney stones, blood dyscrasias, metabolic acidosis, electrolyte imbalance [16].

The oldest antiglaucoma drugs, the parasympathomimetics, have a lot of ocular side effects, such as: miosis, ciliary spasm, stinging, burning, tearing, conjunctival thickening, iris cysts, cataract, pseudomyopia, retinal detachment, and increased pupillary block. The most important systemic effects of pilocarpine and similar drugs are bronchocostriction and intestinal cramp [16].

THE PRESERVATIVES

Beyond therapeutical benefit, all drugs have side effects on various body tissues and functions, also the eye can be affected. IOP-lowering molecules include, besides the active principle, vehicle and preservative. All can be responsible for local and systemic side effects, but while the active agents are fundamental for the treatment of the disease and their side effects have been studied for years, preservatives are not supposed to be dangerous and it is also difficult to avoid using them [17]. The mechanisms responsible for preservatives side effects are not fully understood [18-19], but it is well known that preservatives induce in 90% of cases a toxic reaction and rarely an allergic reaction [20]. The multi-dose topical ophthalmic drugs require a preservative systems against microbial contamination. Even when preserved with benzalkonium chloride (BAK), microbial contamination has been found to be present in 28% to 29% of in-use containers, with a significantly greater frequency in those used for more than 8 weeks [21]. This contamination translated into a high concordance of the same organisms cultured from the conjunctiva, especially in patients with ocular surface disease; one-third of patients reported having touched their eyes during medication installation [22].

The presence of the preservative is useful to decrease potential of ocular infection in case of prolonged usage, but it is well known the side effects on ocular tissues due to a chronic exposure to some preservatives. Preservatives are also important to prevent decomposition of active drug which it will go bad in 1 or 2 weeks in a multidose solutions used twice daily [23].

- Benzalkonium chloride

In over 70% of the ophthalmic multidose containers [24] the preservatives used is benzalkonium chloride. BAK, a quaternary ammonium compound, promotes activation of lipooxygenases and synthesis and secretion of eicosanoids, inflammatory mediators, and many cytokines such as interleukin (IL)-la, IL-8, IL-10 and tumor necrosis factor-α, resulting in delayed hypersensibility and allergic reactions [25]. It has already been found that this compound has a cytotoxic effects on the ocular surface and trabecular meshwork cells [26]. Three mechanisms of BAK toxicity have been described: 1) a detergent effect causing loss of tear film stability, 2) direct damage to the corneal and conjunctival epithelium and 3) immunoallergic reaction [27].

Probably, because of persistence of BAK in cell membranes, the toxicity is delayed and prolonged. The reasons of BAK side effects are the high penetrating capacity [27]. In the past BAK is thought to be essential as ocular penetration enhancer for topically administered drugs, because it increases the corneal permeability of pharmacologic agents [28]. Nowadays, the concept that preservative is necessary for penetration of principle active through cornea is called into question. For example, Pellinen and Lokkila have demonstrated that the penetration into rabbit anterior chamber after topical application of tafluprost 0.0015% eye drops preserved with 0.01% BAK and preservative-free tafluprost 0.0015% was comparable. They concluded that BAK at the concentration used in the tafluprost formulations did not affect corneal penetration of this drug into rabbit aqueous humor. It is possible that tafluprost has its own high corneal penetrating ability and BAK would not enhance it [29].

The toxic effects of BAK depending on the dose and duration of exposure [30]. In multidose bottles BAK is used at an average concentration of 0.01% (range 0.004% –0.02%) [31] and the half-life of BAK from corneal epithelium and conjunctival tissue is 20 hours [32]. In 1999 De Saint Jean et al studied the effect of different concentrations of BAK (0.1– 0.0001%) applied for 10 minutes on a human conjunctival cell line. Exposure to 0.1% and 0.05% BAK caused immediate cell lysis, while exposure to 0.01% BAK was associated with cell death within 24 hours, and doses of 0.005–0.0001% induced apoptotic cell death at 72 hours in a dose-dependent manner [25].

Nowadays it is well known that the preservative BAK has negative effects on the ocular surface: tear film, conjunctiva, cornea [33].

The tear film has an important function in protecting, lubricating and providing trophic factors to the ocular surface. The etiopathogenetic classification of tear film dysfunction separates between aqueous-deficient dry eye and evaporative dry eye. Several factors are causes of extrinsic evaporative dry eye including also the action of toxic topical agents such as preservatives [34]. The tear film is reported to be composed of three layers: lipid, aqueous and mucin layers. A change of any of these layers can result in a tear film dysfunction, due to an inappropriate functions of the tears [35]. The lipid layer provides the air-tear film interface and forms the water vapor barrier that retards evaporation of water from the ocular surface

[36]. In the tear film, the presence of the mucin layer converts the corneal epithelium from a hydrophobic to a hydrophilic surface so that the aqueous tear film can be spread over the cornea. The mucin, produced by the goblet cells throughout the conjunctiva, helps the cornea to hold the tear film on its surface [37]. If the production of mucus is reduced (e.g.: due to goblet cell damage or age), mucus distribution over the preocular surface is impaired, leading to poor contact of the tear film with the eye surface and a loss of film stability [38]. An increase of evaporation and a consequent instability of the tear film are directly caused by BAK. Several studies demonstrated the detergent effect on the pre-corneal film of this preservative [39,40]. Both Herreras et al in 1992 [11] and Arici et al in 2000 [41] showed a statistically significant (P < 0.01) reduction in break-up time (BUT) and Schirmer's test. Herreras et al showed that between the patients who used preserved topical timolol, for an average of 25 months at least, 66% had a pathologic Schirmer's test and 95% a reduction in break-up time (BUT) [11].

The prevalence of tear film dysfunction in patients with glaucoma using topical IOP lowering therapy is recently described in literature and ranges from 48.4% [42] to 59% [43] by using the OSDI questionnaire. Recently, Valente et al [44] found that 52% of patients in therapy with preserved antiglaucomatous drops had symptoms of tear film dysfunction with a positive OSDI. Between all signs of ocular surface, the lissamine green conjunctival staining seemed to be greater in patients using more drops during the day. Symptoms correlated to signs only in patients in monotherapy with β-blockers drops. A therapy with β-blockers was worse for the ocular surface than the others types of glaucoma treatments. The explanation might be that topical timolol treatment, acting also in a systemic way, was responsible of a reduction in tear production [45]. Therefore β-blockers directly damaged the ocular surface as result of the toxicity of preserved drops and indirectly decreasing tear production from lacrimal gland [44]. Another recent study showed that the use of preserved IOP-lowering drugs was often correlated to some clinical symptoms of the ocular surface such as discomfort upon instillation, dry eye, burning, stinging, and foreign body sensation. In particularly, the author found that the use of more antiglaucomatous BAK-containing eyedrops was significantly associated with a higher prevalence of abnormal results on the lissamine green test of the conjunctiva [43].

Arici et al found that in glaucoma patients treated with preserved topical drugs, there were a reduced number of goblet cells on impression cytology responsible of an impaired mucus layer of the tear film [41]. Benzalkonium chloride in fact acts indirectly on the tear film by decreasing the density of goblet cells in the conjunctival epithelium [46,47].

Conjunctival inflammation with an increase of macrophages, lymphocytes and fibroblasts, squamous metaplasia with loss of goblet cells, subconjunctival fibrosis in the conjunctiva and Tenon's capsule are all the result of long-term preserved antiglaucomatous drug use. Many histopathological and impression cytology studies [48-49] confirmed these conjunctival changes caused by BAK. In glaucomatous patients treated with preservatives drugs, Baudolin et al observed a significant increase of immuno-inflammatory markers of the conjunctival epithelium compared with healthy controls [50].

It is well known how the inflammation of the conjunctiva, caused by a topical antiglaucoma therapy, is responsible of a decrease chances of a good outcome of filtration surgery. Young et al. showed an increase in myofibroblastic cell proliferation in fistolized rabbit conjunctiva treated with glaucoma medications or a preserved artificial tear drop compared with untreated controls [51]. Lavin et al. found that filtering surgery was more successful in patients who had received preoperative topical hypotensive drugs for a shorter time (average of 2 weeks). The failure rate of trabeculectomy was significantly correlated to long term (> 1 year) topical antiglaucoma therapy (p < 0.001) [52]. Broadway et al followed, for at least 6 months, 124 patients underwent filtration surgery. They divided the subjects of the study in four groups according to the type of preservatives antiglaucoma treatments used. Patients of group 1 taking minimal topical therapy (who underwent planned primary trabeculectomy within 6 weeks after diagnosis of glaucoma), patients of group 2 receiving beta-blockers, patients of group 3 taking beta-blockers and miotics, patients of group 4 receiving beta-blockers, miotics and sympathomimetics (prostaglandin analogues were not on the marketing yet). In these groups the surgery outcome was 90% (group 1), 93% (group 2), 72% (group 3) and 45% (group 4). The trabeculectomy success rate for patients treated with β-blockers and miotics (group 3) was significantly lower (72%, P<0.01), and that for the group treated with β-blockers, miotics and sympathomimetics (group 4) was even lower (45%, P<0.001). According to these results the authors speculated that the changes of the conjunctiva, resulting in postoperative wound healing and fibrosis, were more significant if more than one drug was administered because of the higher degree of exposure to preservatives. This fibrosis, together with inflammatory infiltrates and cytokine release, plays a role in postoperative fibrotic scarring reaction and therefore contributes to surgical failure [53].

The cornea, together with the conjunctiva, allows the absorption of the drugs.

Any change in tear film composition can cause corneal epithelial cell damage and punctuate epithelial keratitis [54]. In 2001, corneal microlesions covering nearly 9% of the surface were described on a rabbit model after a 28 days treatment with beta-blockers preserved in BAK 0.01% [55]. In another study on rabbit, Dormans et al found after application of 0.01% BAK solution epithelial changes such as complete loss of microvilli, degenerative membrane changes and desquamation of the two superficial epithelial cell layers after an exposure of three hours, by using the scanning electron microscopy [56]. The use of preservatives inhibits corneal cell proliferation and growth [57]. Therefore, corneal healing is impaired [58] and the epithelial barrier is compromised as demonstred by De Jong et al. in 1994. He showed a significant decrease in corneal epithelial permeability (p = 0.025) and a significant increase in corneal autofluorescence (p = 0.003) in 21 glaucomatous patients during treatment with timolol preserved with BAK at concentrations of 0.25% or 0.5% [59].

Baudolin et al explained that an instable tear film interferes with surface wet ability leading to dry eye symptoms, corneal damage and inflammation with production of cytotoxic inflammatory mediators throughout the ocular surface [60]. Two chemokine receptors CCR4 and CCR5 were found over-expressed [61] and the human leukocyte antigen DR (HLA-DR), the intercellular adhesion molecule-1 (ICAM-1) were both significantly higher in patients treated with antiglaucoma drugs [62,63].

Recently in glaucomatous patients with chronic treatment, the use of confocal microscopy has showed ocular surface alterations. Martone et al showed in the group of patients treated with preservative medication a reduction in density of superficial epithelial, an increase in density of basal epithelial cells, a stromal keratocyte activation and changes of sub-basal nerves, more tortuose and lower in number. It is interesting how the reduced number of nerves and the increased tortuosity of sub-basal fibers was correlated with corneal hypoesthesia and reduced tear secretion in the glaucoma therapy groups [64].

Besides affecting the ocular surface, preservatives may also damage trabecular and epithelial lens cells. BAK has a cytotoxic effects on trabecular meshwork cells inhibiting their proliferation at a concentration of 0.00002% in vitro models [65]. Trabecular cells apoptosis should be caused by BAK because the betaxolol preserved with 0.0001% BAK showed a moderate proapoptotic effect, whereas unpreserved betaxolol did not display any apoptosis [66]. Preservatives can also modify the proliferation of epithelial lens cells in fact Goto et al. showed that BAK-containing latanoprost or timolol medications increase lesser than BAK alone the secretion of chemical mediators causing wound healing in a human lens epithelial cell line [67].

In the past there was the doubt that IOP-lowering drugs can accelerate cataract formation [68-69], recently some studies such as the Barbados Eye Study, the Early Manifest Glaucoma Trial and the Collaborative Normal Tension Glaucoma study, confirmed the increased risk of development of nuclear cataract [70-71]. Moreover, the Ocular Hypertension Treatment Study showed an increase of cataract extraction and cataract/filtration surgery in patients treating medically compared with the control group (hazard ratio 1.56, 95% CI confidence interval) [72].

Cystoid macular edema in both pseudophakic patients and aphakic patients is another ocular damage caused by topical hypotensive medications, in particularly non selective adrenergic agonists, beta-blockers and especially prostaglandin analogs. This ocular adverse event in pseudophakic eye can occurs with a posterior lens capsule rupture or in case of a breakdown of the blood-retinal barrier that it is known to be a risk factor for the onset of cystoids macular edema [73]. Miyake et al showed a higher incidence of cystoid macular edema after cataract surgery in patients in therapy with preserved timolol compared with preservative-free timolol [74]. According to Miyake and Ibaraki the preservative rather than the active component of prostaglandin drugs is the causative factor of cystoids macular edema [75]. The incidence of this adverse event should be increased by the presence of the preservatives in the antiglaucoma drops.

Uveitis, with anterior chamber reaction, can occur after a therapy with prostaglandin and it seems to be caused by an alteration of the blood–aqueous barrier [76]. In an objective study of the aqueous flare comparing latanoprost with travoprost and bimatoprost, the travoprost (p < 0.013) and the bimatoprost groups (p < 0.001) had less flare than the latanoprost group after 3 months and also after 6 months of treatment. This is probably explained by a lightly superior break of the blood–aqueous barrier induced by latanoprost [77].

- Alternative of combo medication

Combo medication have been introduced in clinics to improve patients' compliance decreasing the number of drops using daily. At the same time they allow to decrease the local side effects of preservatives included in some formulation of combo medications. Ammar and Kahook evaluated the effects of two combinations (timolol-brimonidine and timolol-dorzolamide) on human ocular surface and found that even if the preservative concentration was reduced because of the less number of drops; both combinations demonstrated a significant reduction in the percentage of live corneal and conjunctival epithelial cells compared with control. Furthermore the difference found between the two medications could be related to the different pH of the drops [78].

All the fixed combinations of anti-glaucomatous drugs in the market contain 0.5% timolole maleate, which has been combined with prostaglandin analogs such as latanoprost (Xalacom®), travoprost (Duotrav®) and bimatoprost (Ganfort ®), with alpha2-agonists such as brimonidine (Combigan ®) and topical carbonic anhidrase inhibitors such as dorzolamide (Cosopt®) and brinzolamide (Azarga®) [79].

A randomized study comprising over 500 patients has demonstrated that this combination is more efficient than each component [80].

- Advantage of alternative preservatives in glaucomatous drops

Besides BAK, there are others alternative preservatives with lower toxicity used in glaucoma formulation: Purite®, sofZia®, Polyquad®.

Purite® is a stabilized oxychloro complex and it is converted in the eye into natural tear components (sodium and chloride ions, oxygen, and water). It belongs to the Category II, mild eye irritant, according to the Environmental Protection Agency. In an animal study [81] thirty eyes of 15 rabbits were randomized to 1 of 6 treatment groups: artificial tears (Refresh Tears, carboxymethyl cellulose 0.5%) BID, brimonidine Purite® 0.15% BID, bimatoprost 0.03% QD, dorzolamide 2% BID, timolol maleate 0.5% BID, or latanoprost 0.005% QD for 30 days. Corneal damage was evaluated by scanning electron microscopy and conjunctival inflammation with light microscopy. After one month of treatment those eyes treated with glaucoma medications containing higher levels of benzalkonium chloride (BAK) had greater corneal damage and conjunctival cell infiltration than the eyes treated with medications preserved with lower levels of BAK or with Purite®.

An alternative preservative system, sofZia®, an ionic buffer that contains borate, sorbitol, propylene glycol and zinc [82], recently has been developed and approved by the U.S. Food and Drug Administration and also in Europe. SofZia has been used since as an alternative to BAK (0.015%) in Travatan Z®, another available formulation of travoprost ophthalmic solution. Recently Kahook and Noecker studied on the rabbits the changes in the number of goblet cells after 30 days of once-daily topical application of latanoprost preserved with 0.02% BAK eye drops (Xalatan®), travoprost preserved with sofZia® eye drops (Travatan Z®), or preservative-free artificial tears. They demonstrated that the number of goblet cells in the latanoprost with BAK group was significantly lower than in the other two groups (p = 0.0001) [83]. When they evaluated corneal epithelial changes by transmission electron microscopy and conjunctival inflammation by light microscopy after hematoxylin and eosin staining, after once-daily dosing, travoprost with sofZia produced significantly (P = 0.0001) less corneal changes and less conjunctival inflammation than latanoprost preserved with BAK. Corneal and conjunctival changes found with travoprost with sofZia were similar to those induced by preservative-free artificial tears [84]. Horsley and Kahook found a measurable improvement from BAK preserved prostaglandin (PGA) to travoprost with sofZia in BUT, corneal staining and OSDI [85]. Moreover, Yamazaki S et al showed an improvement superficial punctate keratopathy switching treatment with latanoprost to SofZia-preserved travoprost [86].

On the other hand, Ryan G Jr at al showed how the presence of BAK 0.02% in Latanoprost formulation compared to travoprost with sofZia provides a more protective environment in the event of contamination and subsequent exposure to microorganisms during use [87]. Recent studies in which patients were videotaped to assess their success at instillation of topical ocular hypotensive medications highlight the concerns about bottle contamination, that it is a more important issue than previously believed [88,89].

In the first of these studies, 92.8% of patients with a diagnosis of glaucoma or ocular hypertension who used 1 or more glaucoma medications for at least 6 months reported no problems administering their eye medications; yet, less than a third of patients were successful at instilling a single drop with touching the bottle to the eye [15]. In a subsequent study in patients with visual impairment or moderate to severe visual field loss, only 39% were able to instill a single drop without touching the eye; age (<70 vs ≥70 years) was found to be a significant predictor for less successful instillation [16]. In summary, use a preservative with low toxicity compared to BAK seems better to improve patient's therapy compliance, but clinicians have to teach to the patients how to put drops into the eye without touching the lids.

Another preservative with lower toxicity compare to BAK is Polyquad®. It is a detergent, derived from BAK. Bacterial cells attract Polyquad, yet human corneal epithelial cells tend to repel the compound [90]. While Polyquad has been shown to be much less toxic to the corneo–conjunctival surface than BAK, [91] it has been shown to cause superficial epithelial damage to the cornea [92]. The main detriment associated with polyquaternium-1 is its tendency to reduce the density of conjunctival goblet cells, thereby decreasing aqueous tear film production [91]. A recent study has evaluated on a rabbit model the toxicity of a novel formulation of fixed-combination travoprost 0.004%/timolol 0.5% ophthalmic solution, which contains the antimicrobial preservative polyquaternium-1 (PQ). The use of this preservative showed a lower ocular surface toxicity compared with the commercial formulation of fixed combinations travoprost 0.004%/timolol 0.5% ophthalmic solution and latanoprost 0.005%/timolol 0.5% ophthalmic solution, which both contain the preservative BAK [93].

The recent emergence of oxidizing preservatives (such as sofZia and Purite) portend a future movement away from detergent preservatives (such as BAK and BAK-derived) and a renewed interest in the deleterious effects manifested in the eye as a consequence of chronic treatments. Industry will continue to seek out newer agents that will preserve medications in multidose bottles while causing fewer side effects on corneal and conjunctival tissues [94].

- Advantage of free-preservatives formulation

Baudolin [95] and Pisella et al [96] analyzed the clinical benefits of the use of preservative-free antiglaucoma treatments. In both studies all symptoms were significantly higher in patients using preserved therapy compared with those using preservative-free drugs. Moreover, all symptoms and signs improved after switching patients to a preservative-free therapy or lighter preservative-containing medicaments. In a comparative retrospective study, with the use of confocal microscopy, the long-term effects of preservative-free and preservative-containing antiglaucoma eye drops were evaluated on the tear secretion and ocular surface. Also in this case, all the clinical scores (corneal sensitivity, Schirmer I test, and lachrymal film break-up time) were significantly lower in the preservative medication groups than in the preservative-free group ($P < 0.05$) [64]. Hence, the new formulations of preservative-free B-blockers and prostaglandin could become an additional therapeutic advantage in what concerns ocular toxicity compared to traditional IOP-lowering drugs associated with benzalkonium chloride. These preservative-free drops have the same effectiveness to maintain IOP at the right level compared to preserved therapy and they allow improvement in quality of life, patient's satisfaction and drop comfort [97].

DISCUSSION

We have analyzed the effects of preserved antiglaucoma drugs on the ocular tissues. Exams to evaluate tear film functions like Schirmer's test, break-up time should be done especially in those patients who have symptoms of dry eye. Conjunctival and corneal epithelia changes using fluorescein and lissamine green staining, measuring of immuno-inflammatory markers and mediators of the inflammations, using impression cytology, should be done in glaucoma clinics to improve the success rate of medical treatment (compliance and adherence) and glaucoma surgery. While the local and systemic side effect of the active agents can be stop changing the therapy, the adverse actions of the preservatives are very difficult to avoid. One possibility to reduce preservatives effects is to use fixed combinations. They assure a reduction in the number of drops instilled per day and a consequence decrease of preservative applied to the eye with its side effects [95]. Moreover they offer convenience saving money and time. Another way to decrease the damage on the ocular tissue caused by BAK, the common preservatives in glaucoma medications, is to use alternative preservatives with a lighter toxicity. Other possibility is to use preservative free medication that should improve the compliance and adherence of the patient. The switch from a preservative-containing to preservative-free drugs, when it is possible, may improve the tolerability of drugs with a lower rate of discontinuation and a better adherence to the glaucomatous treatment. Nowadays and surely more in the future, new reformulations of existing products with a better tolerability and a lighter toxicity or in a preservative free formulation are and will be to work out.

It is well known that the preoperative preparation of the eye is now believed essential to improve all surgery outcomes, including glaucoma surgery. A long term topical drug combination is associated with a higher risk of external scarring of the bleb which is the main cause of surgery failure [98]. To improve outcome of filtering surgery, it is necessary to reduce preoperative conjunctival inflammation due to a long term exposure to preservative antiglaucoma medications. Thus, to prepare the eye to a better result after filtering surgery, we should stop some of topical antiglaucoma drugs. It has been suggested that miotics, known to break down the blood-aqueous barrier, should be discontinued at least 2 weeks before surgery [99]. Moreover we should use preservative-free therapy that we showed to have a less impact on ocular tissues. Also the addition of preoperative topical corticosteroid therapy or anti-inflammatory eye drops helps to increase the success rate of filtering surgery, decreasing in inflammation of the conjunctiva at the time of surgery. Broadway et al tried to reverse conjunctival changes in the immediate preoperative period in 30 patients who were receiving multiple antiglaucoma medications. These patients underwent an inferior bulbar conjunctival biopsy to detect the number of fibroblasts and the degree of inflammation, then they ceased the sympathomimetic drops, and began treatment with topical corticosteroid (1% fluorometholone) four times daily during the month before the surgery. After one month there was a decrease in inflammatory cells through the conjunctiva and so this preoperative therapy may have improved the success rate of trabeculectomy [100]. It is well known the potential intraocular hypertensive effects of steroids. Probably this was the reason that has brought Baudolin et al to study the efficacy and safety of non-steroidal anti-inflammatory eye drops on the decrease of conjunctival inflammation, following chronic antiglaucoma drugs, in comparison with a steroidal ophthalmic solution. In this study two treatments, preservative-free indomethacin 0.1% and preserved fluorometholone, were given to the two groups of patients on the basis of 1 drop 4 times daily for 1 month before filtering surgery. Patients did not stop the antiglaucoma drugs used for at least 3 years. Conjunctival impression assessed the percentage of cells expressing HLA-DR at the baseline and after 30 days. At the end of the study the percentage of cells expressing HLA-DR had significantly decreased in both treatment groups: the mean reduction was 29.7% from a baseline value of 51.4% in the indomethacin group (P=0.02) and 32.5% from a baseline value of 48.7% in the fluorometholone group (P<0.001). Both anti-inflammatory eye-drops were effective in reducing subclinical conjunctival inflammation before filtering surgery without any significant difference between groups [101].

By confocal microscopy and anterior segment optical coherence tomography, several ocular effects of topical long-term glaucoma medications could be better visualized in the future.

REFERENCES

[1]   Thylefors DS, Negrel AD, Pararajasegaram R, Dadzie KY. Global data on blindness. *Bull World Health Organ.*73, 115–21 (1995).

[2]   Quigley HA. Number of people with glaucoma worldwide. *Br. J. Ophthalmol.* 80(5), 389-93 (1996).

[3]   Quigley HA. Glaucoma. *Lancet.* 16;377(9774):1367-77 (2011).

[4]   Congdon N, O'Colmain B, Klaver CC, et al. Causes and prevalence of visual impairment among adults in the United States. *Arch. Ophthalmol.* 122:477–85 (2004).

[5]   Miglior S, Torri V, Zeyen T, et al. European Glaucoma Prevention Study (EGPS) Group. Intercurrent factors associated with the development of open-angle glaucoma in the European Glaucoma Prevention Study. *Am. J. Ophthalmol.* 144(2): 266–275 (2007).

[6]   Bengtsson B, Leske MC, Hyman L, Heijl A. Fluctuation of intraocular pressure and glaucoma progression in the Early Manifest Glaucoma Trial. *Ophthalmology.* 114(2):205–209 (2007).

[7]   Mush DC, Gillespie BW, Niziol LM, et al. Factors associated with intraocular pressure before and during 9 years of treatment in the Collaborative Initial Glaucoma Treatment Study. *Ophthalmology.* 115(6):927–933 (2008).

[8]   The AGIS Investigators. The Advanced Glaucoma Intervention Study (AGIS): 12. Baseline risk factors for sustained loss of visual field and visual acuity in patients with advanced glaucoma. *Am. J. Ophthalmol.* 134(4):499–512 (2002).

[9]   Lindblom B, Nordmann JP, Sellem E, et al. A multicentre, retrospective study of resource utilization and costs associated with glaucoma management in France and Sweden. *Acta Ophthalmol. Scand.* 84, 74–83 (2006).

[10] Pisella PJ, Pouliquen P, Baudouin C. Prevalence of ocular symptoms and signs with preserved and preservative-free glaucoma medication. *Br. J. Ophthalmol.* 86, 418–423 (2002).

[11] Jaenen N, Baudouin C, Pouliquen P, et al. Ocular symptoms and signs with preserved and preservative-free glaucoma medications. *Eur. J. Ophthalmol.* 17, 341–349 (2007).

[12] Hommer A. A review of preserved and preservative-free prostaglandin analogues for the treatment of open-angle glaucoma and ocular hypertension. *Drugs Today (Barc).* 46(6):409-16 (2010).

[13] Renieri G, Führer K, Scheithe K, et al. Efficacy and tolerability of preservative-free eye drops containing a fixed combination of dorzolamide and timolol in glaucoma patients. *J. Ocul. Pharmacol. Ther.* 26(6):597-603 (2010).

[14] Van der Valk R, Webers CAB, Schouten JSAG, et al. Intraocular pressure-lowering effects of all commonly used glaucoma drugs: a meta-analysis of randomized clinical trials. *Ophthalmology.* 112(7):1177-85 (2005).

[15] European Glaucoma Society. Terminology and Guidelines for Glaucoma III Edition. 122-126 (2008).

[16] European Glaucoma Society. Terminology and Guidelines for Glaucoma III Edition. 127-137 (2008).

[17] Valente C, Iester M. Impact of glaucoma medication on ocular tissue. *Expert Rev. Ophthalmol.* 5(3): 405– 412 (2010).

[18] Herreras JM, Pastor JC, Calonge M, Asensio VM. Ocular surface alteration after long-term treatment with an antiglaucomatous drug. *Ophthalmology.* 99, 1082–8 (1992).

[19] Derous D, De Keizer W, De Wolff-Rouendall D, Soudjin W. Conjunctival keratinisation, an abnormal reaction to an ocular beta-blocker. *Acta Ophthalmol. Scand.* 67, 333–8 (1989).

[20] Wilson FM. Adverse external ocular effects of topical ophthalmicmedications. *Surv Ophthalmol.* 24, 57–88 (1979).

[21] Geyer O, Bottone EJ, Podos SM, et al. Microbial contamination of medications used to treat glaucoma. *Br. J. Ophthalmol* 79:376-379, (1995).

[22] Schein OD, Hibberd PL, Starck T, et al. Microbial contamination of in-use ocular medications. *Arch. Ophthalmol.* 1992, 110:82-85.

[23] Schein OD, Hibberd PL, Starck T, et al. Microbial contamination of in-use ocular medications. *Arch. Ophthalmol.* 110, 82–85 (1992).

[24] Freeman PD, KahooK MY. Preservatives in topical ophthalmic medications: historical and clinical perspectives. *Expert Rev. Ophthalmol.* 4(1), 59-64 (2009).

[25] De Saint Jean M, Brignole F, Bringuier AF, et al. Effects of benzalkonium chloride on growth and survival of Chang conjunctival cells. *Invest Ophthalmol. Vis. Sci.* 40, 619–630 (1999).

[26] de Saint JM, Debbasch C, Brignole F, et al. Toxicity of preserved and unpreserved antiglaucoma topical drugs in an vitro model of conjunctival cells. *Curr. Eye Res.* 20(2):85–94 (2000).

[27] Yee RW. The effect of drop vehicle on the efficacy and side effects of topical glaucoma therapy: a review. *Curr. Opin. Ophthalmol.* 18,134 –139 (2007).

[28] Debbasch C, De Saint JM, Pisella PJ, et al. Quaternary ammonium cytotoxicity in a human conjunctival cell line. *J. Fr. Ophtalmol.* 22, 950–8 (1999).

[29] Thygesen J. In search of improved prostaglandin treatment for glaucoma. *Acta Ophthalmol.* 86 Suppl 242:S5–S6 (2008).

[30] Pellinen P, Lokkila J. Corneal penetration into rabbit aqueous humor is comparable between preserved and preservative-free tafluprost. *Ophthalmic Res.* 41(2):118–122 (2009).

[31] Baudouin C, Pisella PJ, Fillacier K, et al. Ocular surface inflammatory changes induced by topical antiglaucoma drugs. Human and animal studies. *Ophthalmology.* 106, 556 – 563 (1999).

[32] Pisella PJ, Fillacier K, Elena PP, et al. Comparison of the effects of preserved and unpreserved formulations of timolol on the ocular surface of albino rabbits. *Ophthalmic Res.* 32, 3–8 (2000).

[33] Kuppens EVMJ, de Jong CA, Stolwijk TR, et al. Effect of timolol with and without preservative on the basal tear turnover in glaucoma. *Br. J. Ophthalmol.* 79, 339–42 (1995).

[34] Lemp M.A. The definition and classification of dry eye disease: report of the International Dry Eye Workshop (DEWS) *The Ocular Surface.* 5(2): 75-92, (2007).

[35] Rolando M, Zierhut M. The ocular surface and tear film and their dysfunction in dry eye disease. *Surv. Ophthalmol.* 45 Suppl 2:S203-10 (2001).

[36] McCulley JP, Shine WE. The lipid layer of tears: dependent on meibomian gland function. *Exp. Eye Res.* 78, 361-365 (2004).

[37] Lemp MA, Holly FJ, Iwata S, Dohlman CH. The precorneal tear film. I. Factors in spreading and maintaining a continuous tear film over the corneal surface. *Arch. Ophthalmol.* 83(1), 89-94 (1970).

[38] Paulsen F, Langer G, Hoffmann W, Berry M. Human lacrimal gland mucins. *Cell Tissue Res.* 316, 167-177 (2004).

[39] Burstein NL. The effects of topical drugs and preservatives on the tears and corneal epithelium in dry eye. *Trans. Ophthalmol. Soc. UK.* 104, 402–409 (1985).

[40] Baudouin C, de Lunardo C. Short term comparative study of topical 2% carteolol with and without benzalkonium chloride in healthy volunteers. *Br. J. Ophthalmol.* 82, 39–42 (1998).

[41] Arici MK, Arici DS, Topalkara A, Güler C. Adverse effects of topical antiglaucoma drugs on the ocular surface. *Clin. Experiment Ophthalmol.* 28(2), 113-7 (2000).

[42] Fechtner RD, Godfrey DG, Budenz D, et al. Prevalence of ocular surface complaints in patients with glaucoma using topical intraocular pressure-lowering medications. *Cornea.* 29(6):618-21 (2010).

[43] Leung EW, Medeiros FA, Weinreb RN. Prevalence of ocular surface disease in glaucoma patients. *J. Glaucoma.* 17(5), 350-5 (2008).

[44] Valente C, Iester M, Corsi E, Rolando M. Symptoms and Signs of Tear Film Dysfunction in Glaucomatous Patients. *J. Ocul. Pharmacol. Ther* 27(3):2281-285 (2011).

[45] Bonomi L, Zavarise G, Noya E, et al. Effects of timolol maleate on tear flow in human eyes. *Albrecht. Von. Graefes. Arch. Klin. Exp. Ophthalmol.* 213(1):19-22 (1980).

[46] Yalvaç IS, Gedikoğlu G, Karagöz Y, et al. Effect of antiglaucoma drugs on ocular surface. *Acta Ophthalmol. Scand.* 73, 248–56 (1995).

[47] Rolando M, Brezzo V, Giordano G. In: van Bijsterveld OP, Lemp MA, Spinelli D, eds. Symposium on the lacrimal system - Singapore 1990. Amsterdam: Kugler and Ghedini. 87–91 (1991).

[48] Mietz H, Niesen U, Krieglstein GK. The effect of preservatives and antiglaucomatous medication on the histopathology of the conjunctiva. *Graefes Arch. Clin. Exp. Ophthalmol.* 232, 561–5 (1994).

[49] Baun O, Heegaard S, Kessing SV, Prause JU. The morphology of conjunctiva after long term topical anti-glaucoma treatment. *Acta Ophthalmol. Scand.* 73, 242–245 (1995).

[50] Baudouin C, Liang H, Hamard P, et al. The ocular surface of glaucoma patients treated over the longterm expresses inflammatory markers related to both T-helper 1 and T-helper 2 pathways. *Ophthalmology.* 115, 109–115 (2008).

[51] Young TL, Higginbotham EJ, Zou X, Farber MD. Effect of topical glaucoma drugs on fistulized rabbit conjunctiva. *Ophthalmology.* 97, 1423–7 (1990).

[52] Lavin MJ, Wormald RPL, Migdal CS, Hitchings RA. The influence of prior therapy on the success of trabeculectomy. *Arch. Ophthalmol.* 108, 1543–8 (1990).

[53] Broadway DC, Grierson I, O'Brien C, Hitchings RA. Adverse effect of antiglaucoma medication: II. The outcome of filtration surgery. *Arch. Ophthalmol.* 112, 1446–54 (1994).

[54] International Dry Eye Workshop (DEWS). *The Ocular Surface.* 5(2) (2007).

[55] Furrer P, Berger J, Mayer JM, Gurny R. A comparative study of the ocular tolerance of three timolol-based preparations: the influence of preservatives on ocular tolerance. *J. Fr. Ophtalmol.* 24, 13–19 (2001).

[56] Dormans JA, Van Logten MJ. The effects of ophthalmic preservatives on corneal epithelium of the rabbit: a scanning electron microscopical study. *Toxicol. Appl. Pharmacol.* 62, 251–61 (1982).

[57] Samples JR, Binder PS, Nayak S. The effect of epinephrine and benzalkonium chloride on cultured corneal endothelial and trabecular meshwork cells. *Exp. Eye Res.* 49, 1–12 (1989).

[58] Grant RL, Acosta D. Prolonged adverse effects of benzalkonium chlorideand sodium dodecyl sulfate in a primary culture system of rabbit corneal epithelial cells. *Fundam Appl. Toxicol.* 33, 71–82 (1996).

[59] De Jong C, Stolwijk T, Kuppens E, et al. Topical timolol with and without benzalkonium chloride: epithelial permeability and autofluorescence of the cornea in glaucoma. *Graefes Arch. Clin. Exp. Ophthalmol.* 232, 221–224 (1994).

[60] Baudouin C. The pathology of dry eye. *Surv. Ophthalmol.* 45(2), 211–220 (2001).

[61] Costagliola C, Prete AD, Incorvaia C, et al. Ocular surface changes induced by topical application of latanoprost and timolol: a short-term study in glaucomatous patients with and without allergic conjunctivitis. *Graefes Arch. Clin. Exp. Ophthalmol.* 239, 809–814 (2001).

[62] Pisella PJ, Debbasch C, Hamard P, et al. Conjunctival proinflammatory and proapoptotic effects of latanoprost and preserved and unpreserved timolol: an ex vivo and in vitro study. *Invest. Ophthalmol. Vis. Sci.* 45, 1360–1368 (2004).

[63] Baudouin C, Hamard P, Liang H, et al. Conjunctival epithelial cell expression of interleukins and inflammatory markers in glaucoma patients treated over the longterm. *Ophthalmology.* 111, 2186–2192 (2004).

[64] Martone G, Frezzotti P, Tosi GM, et al. An in vivo confocal microscopy analysis of effects of topical antiglaucoma therapy with preservative on corneal innervation and morphology. *Am. J. Ophthalmol.* 147, 725–735 (2009).

[65] Broadway DC, Grierson I, O'Brien C, et al. Adverse effects of topical antiglaucoma medication. I. The conjunctival cell profile. *Arch. Ophthalmol.* 112, 1437–45 (1994).

[66] Hamard P, Debbasch C, Blondin C, et al. Human trabecular cells and apoptosis: in vitro evaluation of the effect of betaxolol with or without preservative. *J. Fr. Ophtalmol.* 25, 777–784 (2002).

[67] Goto Y, Ibaraki N and Miyake K. Human lens epithelial cell damage and stimulation of their secretion of chemical mediators by benzalkonium chloride rather than latanoprost and timolol. *Arch. Ophthalmol.* 121, 835–839 (2003).

[68] Shaffer RN, Rosenthal G. Comparison of cataract incidence in normal and glaucomatous population. *Am. J. Ophthalmol.* 69(3), 368–370 (1970).

[69] Harding JJ, Egerton M, van Heyningen R, Harding RS. Diabetes, glaucoma, sex, and cataract: analysis of combined data from two case control studies. *Br. J. Ophthalmol.* 77, 2–6 (1993).

[70] Leske MC, Wu SY, Nemesure B, Hennis A. Barbados Eye Studies Group. Risk factors for incident nuclear opacities. *Ophthalmology.* 109, 1303–1308 (2002).

[71] Collaborative normal-tension glaucoma study group. Comparison of glaucomatous progression between untreated patients with normal tension glaucoma and patients with therapeutically reduced intraocular pressure. *Am. J. Ophthalmol.* 126, 487-497 (1998).

[72] Herman DC, Gordon MO, Beiser JA, et al. Topical ocular hypotensive medication and lens opacification: evidence from the Ocular Hypertension Treatment Study. *Am. J. Ophthalmol.* 142, 800–810 (2006).

[73] Miyake K, Ota I, Maekubo K, Ichihashi S, Miyake S. Latanoprost accelerates disruption of the blood-aqueous barrier and the incidence of angiographic cystoid macular edema in early postoperative pseudophakias. *Arch. Ophthalmol.* 117, 34-40 (1999).

[74] Miyake K, Ibaraki N, Goto Y, et al. ESCRS Binkhorst Lecture 2002. Pseudophakic preservative maculopathy. *J. Cataract Refract. Surg.* 29, 1800–1810 (2003).

[75] Miyake K, Ibaraki N. Prostaglandins and cystoid macular edema. *Surv. Ophthalmol.* 47(1), 203-218 (2002).

[76] Ardjomand N, Eckhardt M, Berghold A, Faulborn J et al.Synthesis pattern of matrix metalloproteinases (MMPs) and inhibitors (TIMPs) in human explant organ cultures after treatment with latanoprost and dexamethasone. *Eye.*14, 375–83 (2000).

[77] Cellini M, Caramazza R, Bonsanto D, et al. Prostaglandin analogs and blood-aqueous barrier integrity: a flare cell meter study. *Ophthalmologica.* 218, 312–7 (2004).

[78] Ammar DA, Kahook MY. The effects of combination glaucoma medications on ocular surface epithelial cells. *Adv. Ther.* 26(10), 970-5 (2009).

[79] Muñoz-Negrete FJ, Pérez-López M, Won Kim HR, Rebolleda G. New developments in glaucoma medical treatment. *Arch. Soc. Esp. Oftalmol.* 84(10):491-500 (2009).

[80]   Kaback M, Scoper SV, Arzeno G, et al. Intraocular Pressure-Lowering Efficacy of Brinzolamide 1%/Timolol 0.5% Fixed combination Compared with Brinzolamide 1% and Timolol 0.5%. *Ophthalmology* 115: 1728-1734 (2008).

[81]   Herrygers LA, Anwaruddin R. Corneal and conjunctival changes caused by commonly used glaucoma medications. *Cornea.* 23(5), 490-6 (2004).

[82]   Travatan Z (travoprost ophthalmic solution): US product insert. Alcon laboratories, Fort Worth, TX, 2005-2007 [http://ecatalog.alcon.com/pi/TravatanZ_us_en.pdf].

[83]   Kahook MY, Noecker R Quantitative analysis of conjunctival goblet cells after chronic application of topical drops. *Adv. Ther.* 25, 743–51 (2008).

[84]   Kahook MY, Noecker R. Comparison of corneal and conjunctival changes after dosing of travoprost preserved with sofZia, latanoprost with 0.02% benzalkonium chloride, and preservative-free artificial tears. *Cornea.* 27(3), 339-43 (2008).

[85]   Horsley MB, Kahook MY. Effects of prostaglandin analog therapy on the ocular surface of glaucoma patients. *Clin. Ophthalmol.* 3, 291-5 (2009).

[86]   Yamazaki S, Nanno M, Kimura T, et al. Effects of switching to SofZia-preserved travoprost in patients who presented with superficial punctate keratopathy while under treatment with latanoprost. *Jpn J. Ophthalmol.* 54(1):7-14. (2010).

[87]   Ryan G Jr, Fain JM, Lovelace C, Gelotte KM. Effectiveness of ophthalmic solution preservatives: a comparison of latanoprost with 0.02% benzalkonium chloride and travoprost with the sofZia preservative system. *BMC Ophthalmol.* 21;11(1):8 (2011).

[88]   Stone JL, Robin AL, Novack GD, et al. An objective evaluation of eyedrop instillation in patients with glaucoma. *Arch. Ophthalmol.* 127:732-736. (2009).

[89]   Hennessy AL, Katz J, Covert D, et al. Videotaped evaluation of eyedrop instillation in glaucoma patients with visual impairment or moderate to severe visual field loss. *Ophthalmology* 117:2345-2352 (2010).

[90]   Rosenthal R, Henry C, Stone R, Schlech B. Anatomy of a regimen: consideration of multipurpose solutions during non-compliant use. *Cont. Lens Anterior Eye* 26(1),17–26 (2003).

[91]   Labbé A, Pauly A, Liang H et al. Comparison of toxicological profiles of benzalkonium chloride and polyquaternium-1: an experimental study. *J. Ocul. Pharmacol. Ther.* 22(4),267–278 (2006).

[92]   Lopez B, Ubel J. Quantitative evaluation of the corneal epithelial barrier: effect of artificial tears and preservatives. *Curr. Eye Res.* 10(7),645–656 (1991).

[93]   Liang H, Brignole-Baudouin F, Pauly A, Riancho L, Baudouin C. Polyquad-preserved travoprost/timolol, benzalkonium chloride (BAK)-preserved travoprost/timolol, and latanoprost/timolol in fixed combinations: a rabbit ocular surface study. *Adv. Ther.* 28(4):311-25 (2011).

[94]   Freeman PD, Kahook MY et al. Preservatives in Topical Ophthalmic Medications: Historical and Practical Review of Benzalkonium Chloride. *Expert. Rev. Ophthalmol.* 4(1):59-64 (2009).

[95]   Baudolin C. Detrimental effect of preservatives in eyedrops: implications for the treatment of glaucoma. *Acta Ophthalmol.* 86, 716–726 (2008).

[96]   Pisella PJ, Pouliquen P, Baudouin C. Prevalence of ocular symptoms and signs with preserved and preservative-free glaucoma medication. *Br. J. Ophthalmol.* 86, 418–423 (2002).

[97] Uusitalo H, Chen E, Pfeiffer N, et al. Switching from a preserved to a preservative-free prostaglandin preparation in topical glaucoma medication. *Acta Ophthalmol.* 88(3):329-36 (2010).

[98] Fechtner RD, Realini T. Fixed combinations of topical glaucoma medications. *Current Opinion in Ophthalmology.* 15, 132–135 (2004).

[99] Skuta GL, Parrish RK. II.Wound healing in glaucoma filtering surgery. *Surv Ophthalmol.* 32, 149-170 (1987).

[100] BroadwayDC, Grierson I, Störmer J, Hitchings RA. Reversal of Topical Antiglaucoma Medication Effects on the Conjunctiva. *Arch. Ophthalmol.* 114, 262-267 (1996).

[101] Baudolin C, Nordmann JP, Denis P, et al. Efficacy of indomethacin 0.1% and fluorometholone 0.1% on conjunctival inflammation following chronic application of antiglaucomatous drugs. *Graefe's Arch. Clin. Exp. Ophthalmol.* 240, 929–935 (2002).

In: Glaucoma: Etiology, Pathogenesis and Treatments   ISBN: 978-1-61470-975-6
Editors: Z. G. Fei and S. Zeng   © 2012 Nova Science Publishers, Inc.

Chapter IV

Uveitic Glaucoma

Ester Carreño[1], Alejandro Portero[2], Fernando Ussa[2] and José M. Herreras[1,2]

[1] Hospital Clínico Universitario de Valladolid, Spain
[2] Ocular Immunology Unit-IOBA (Instituto Universitario de Oftalmobiología),
University of Valladolid, Campus Miguel Delibes, Valladolid, Spain

ABSTRACT

Secondary uveitic glaucoma is a common complication of intraocular inflammation and is present in up to 20% of patients with uveitis. The incidence of uveitis in the United States is estimated to be 200 cases per 100 000 people per year and mostly affects adults aged 20 to 50 years. This condition represents the fourth cause of legal blindness in patients between 20 and 60 years. Among the patients with uveitis visual loss occurs more frequently in patients with glaucoma than in patients without glaucoma. Several mechanisms are involved in the pathogenesis of uveitic glaucoma. It is clinically useful to classify it into 4 categories based on mechanism: inflammatory ocular hypertension syndrome; ocular hypertension due to acute uveitic angle closure; corticosteroid-induced ocular hypertension/glaucoma; and ocular hypertension/glaucoma due to chronic damage to aqueous outflow systems, most notably the trabecular meshwork. Uveitic glaucoma often gets worse despite intensive medical treatment, and it may require surgical intervention. Surgical management is challenging because of the increased risk of post-operative inflammation and failure to control intraocular pressure.

INTRODUCTION AND DEFINITION

The incidence of uveitis in the United States is estimated to be 200 cases per 100 000 people per year and mostly affects adults aged 20 to 50 years[1]. This condition represents the fourth cause of legal blindness in patients between 20 and 60 years [1]. Among the patients with uveitis, visual loss occurs more frequently in patients with glaucoma than in patients without glaucomatous neuropathy [2]. Historically the association between uveitis and glaucoma was recognized in the early nineteenth century and the austrian ophthalmologist G.J. Beer has been credited as the first to report in 1813 the association, describing it as "arthritic iritis" with dilatation of the pupil and a gray-green deep obscuration caused by vitreous opacity, followed by glaucoma and blindness [3]. Desmans in 1981, Weller en 1825, and MacKenzie in 1830 also described the association between uveitis and glaucoma[4]. In 1857 Albrecht von Graefe proposed iridectomy for the treatment of acute as well as uveitic glaucoma and reported a series of 20 eyes that underwent successful iridectomy for uveitic glaucoma [5]. In 1877 Adolph Weber proposed the hypothesis of hypersecretion and the presence of an altered aqueous in inflammatory glaucoma [6]. In 1989, P. Smith proposed the first modern classification of uveitic glaucoma [7]. Later, specific types of uveitic glaucoma were described by Fuchs in 1906 (Fuchs' heterochromic uveitis) [8] and Posner and Schlossman in 1948 (glaucomatocyclitic crisis) [9].Secondary glaucoma is properly considered to represent those eyes in which a second form of ocular pathology has caused IOP above the normal range, leading to optic nerve damage [10]. The diagnosis of secondary uveitic glaucoma (also denominated inflammatory glaucoma) is based on the presence of optic neuropathy and in the presence of any kind of uveitis (this definition also includes the steroid-induced glaucoma). There was consensus that the term glaucoma should not be considered synonymous with elevated intraocular pressure (IOP) in a patient with uveitis, but that it should be reserved for those situations where there is either observed glaucomatous disk damage or demonstrated visual field loss. The term elevated IOP should be used for those situations where there is an IOP above a defined normal range or when there is an increase in IOP from baseline during a study with longitudinal data. The threshold for considering a rise in IOP substantial is usually 10 mm Hg or greater. Although consensus was not achieved on the threshold for considering an IOP as elevated, the choices were narrowed to two. The first was to report at two levels: above 21 mm Hg (the traditional "upper limit of normal") and above 30 mm Hg (a level above which many practitioners would initiate treatment even without evidence of glaucomatous damage). The second option was to report IOP above the 24 mm Hg as elevated, as the risk of glaucoma appears to increase substantially as the IOP increases beyond this level [11].

The estimated proportion of glaucoma damage that is clearly secondary (including uveitic, traumatic, neovascular and lens-related glaucoma) to other ocular or systemic disease, or to trauma, may represent as much as 20% of all glaucoma [10].Inflammatory glaucoma occurs in 8% to 26% of patients with acute uveitis and in 11% to 46% of patients with chronic uveitis, and the risk of elevated IOP has been shown to increase over time [2, 12-14].Famous writer James Joyce, was affected by this pathology, even some authors wonder if the Ulysses had been the same if Joyce had not suffer from uveitic glaucoma [15].

CLASSIFICATION

It is clinically useful to classify ocular hypertension in patients with uveitis into 4 categories based on mechanism. These include inflammatory ocular hypertension syndrome (IOHS); ocular hypertension due to acute uveitic angle closure; corticosteroid-induced ocular hypertension/glaucoma; and ocular hypertension/glaucoma due to chronic damage to aqueous outflow systems, most notably the trabecular meshwork.

1. Inflammatory Ocular Hypertension Syndrome

IOHS is defined as an acute and transient increase in IOP in the settings of acute or recurrent inflammation, caused by direct inflammation of the trabecular meshwork, which responds readily to antiinflammatory or/and antimicrobial therapy.

Well-known causes of IOHS include herpetic anterior uveitis and Posner-Schlossman Syndrome [9, 16]. Other less known causes include sarcoid uveitis [17], toxoplasmicretinochoroiditis [18] and syphilitic uveitis [19].

2. Ocular Hypertension due to Acute Uveitic Angle Closure

As with IOHS, this type of secondary ocular hypertension occurs at or near the onset of inflammation. Angle closure may occur in uveitis by a number of mechanisms, such as a result of pupil block secondary to a secluded pupil, synechial closure from iridocorneal contact, an inflammatory or neovascular angle membrane, or forward motion of the iris-lens diaphragm in the presence of a posterior segment space-occupying lesion.

3. Corticosteroid-Induced Ocular Hypertension/Glaucoma

Several agents are capable of inducing an increase in IOP in both normal eyes and eyes with uveitis and/or glaucoma, including topical, periocular, intravitreal and systemic corticosteroids, as well as sustained-release intravitreal implants containing corticosteroid. The extent of IOP elevation depends on the potency of the corticosteroid, the dose and duration of the treatment, the route of administration, and the patient's susceptibility to corticosteroid-induced ocular hypertension [20]. While all corticosteroid administration routes have been associated with elevated IOP [21], local ocular administration is associated with a greater risk, and of local delivery methods, intraocular delivery carries the greater risk, being reported a percentage of 76% of implanted eyes reaching an IOP elevation of 10 mmHg or more from baseline [22]. Typically, corticosteroid-induced ocular hypertension/glaucoma occurs weeks to months after initiating treatment and as such can be readily distinguished from both IOHS and elevated IOP due to acute uveitic angle closure. While the IOP normalizes after cessation of corticosteroid therapy in most cases, ocular hypertension may persist in some patients despite discontinuation of the medication.

4. Hypertension/Glaucoma due to Chronic Damage to Aqueous Outflow Systems

In severe, chronic, or repeated episodes of anterior uveitis, permanent changes in the trabecular meshwork may result in loss or dysfunction of trabecular endothelial cells, scarring of the meshwork or Schlemm's canal, and obstruction of the trabeculum by a hyaline membrane [23].

PATHOPHYSIOLOGY

Elevated IOP in patients with uveitis is relatively common. The mechanism by which this inflammatory process produces an increase of the IOP is multifactorial and poorly understood. Because of the inflammatory status several factors lead to alteration of IOP level.

Depending on the factor the variation will produce an increase or lowering of the IOP. The main responsible factors that may vary the IOP are:

1. Location, nature and duration of the underlying cause of uveitis:

Anterior uveitis is predominantly more frequent in patients with uveitic glaucoma in contrast to intermediate, posterior and panuveitis [12]. Herpes virus-associated uveitis, Fuchs' uveitis, Vogt-Koyanagi-Harada (VKH), syphilis, toxoplasmosis and sarcoidosis were the leading causes of uveitic glaucoma in uveitis adult individuals. On the other hand, Juvenile rheumatoid arthritis (JRA) is the main cause of inflammatory glaucoma in children [12, 24]. Chronic and granulomatous are the characteristics more frequently seen of uveitis, which subsequently lead to uveitic glaucoma. The duration of inflammatory process is also related to the glaucomatous neuropathy, thus chronic and mild symptomatic uveitis have more risk to develop uveitic glaucoma like occurs on JRA in child and Posner-Scholssman syndrome in adults. Both ones can go unnoticed for years destroying gradually the nervous fibers layer.

2. Aqueous production and outflow facility in uveitis:

It is widely believed that elevated IOP in glaucoma is due to the impairment of aqueous outflow through the trabecular meshwork at the juxtacanalicular level and at the inner wall of Schlemm's canal [25]. However, the real mechanism remains unknown by lack of pathology studies in uveitic patients. It is also well known that there are several factors responsible in altering the production, composition and the final outflow of the aqueous humor:

a) Inflammation of the ciliary body usually leads to reduce aqueous production due to its edema and, combined with increased uveoscleral outflow often seen in inflammatory states, hypotony often is a consequence.
b) The trabecular meshwork may be also directly affected by inflammatory insults resulting in reducing outflow. This is frequently seen in herpetic keratouveitis and Posner-Schlossman syndrome where generally produce very high IOP with a mild clinical intraocular identifiable inflammation. In both cases, herpes virus would involve the trabecular meshwork leading to trabecullitis and a subsequently trabecular meshwork edema increasing the outflow resistance and rising the IOP which is characteristic of these entities.
c) Aqueous composition and its production rate: aqueous fluorophotometry studies indicate that aqueous protein arises from ciliary body capillaries in the normal eye. Prevented from entering the aqueous by the ciliary epithelial barrier, protein enters the anterior chamber by the iris stroma and anterior iris surface [26]. In anterior uveitis, however, it is likely that dilated iris and ciliary body vessels account for the increased protein level [27]. The inflamed ciliary body reduces aqueous production

increasing the protein rate of this fluid becoming more viscous. Elevated levels of cytokines in the aqueous humor in patients with uveitis may play an important role in the development of uveitis glaucoma through adverse effects on aqueous outflow facility. However, that increased vascular permeability in uveitis may fail to reverse after resolution of the inflammation leading to chronic elevation of protein rate, which is seen clinically as chronic flare [28]. Furthermore resistance to outflow is believed to vary with the rate of trabecular meshwork perfusion because a trabecular meshwork perfusion rate of less than $1\mu L/min$ may have a deleterious influence on trabecular meshwork function. This process manifests itself clinically in the apparition of spontaneous closure of a cyclodialysis cleft, where a sudden elevation of IOP may occur [29].

d) Mechanical blockage and cellular depletion: pigment and cellular debris may deposit in trabecular meshwork. The phagocytosis of melanin by trabecular meshwork cells leads to trabecular meshwork cell death or depopulation by migration away from that location. Loss of cells from juxtacanalicular meshwork seems to be accompanied by loss of trabecular spaces and an accompanying increase in outflow resistance [30].

3.   Effect of corticosteroid on uveitic glaucoma:

Elevation of IOP 6 to 15 mmHg induced by corticosteroids occurs in about one third of normal individuals and only about 5% having a rise ≥ 15 mmHg[31]. However in patients with Primary open angle glaucoma (POAG) that also have elevated aqueous outflow resistance, 50% of patients suffer a rise of ≥ 15 mmHg. Based on this observation, corticosteroids are likely to have a stronger effect in inducing elevated IOP in patients with a previously compromised outflow pathway [24]. Although there are multiple genes linked to several types of glaucoma, there are not currently reports about a direct association between these genes and uveitic glaucoma. The mechanisms by which steroids may elevate the IOP are multiple and include: alterations in cell size [32], cytoskeletal organization [33], extracellular matrix deposition [34] and matrix metalloproteinasesexpression [35]. All of them increase the outflow resistance of the trabecular meshwork. This effect is very important to keep in mind because corticosteroid regimen is the first and main treatment in uveitic flare-ups. On the other hand, the introduction of immunomodulatory treatments as long-term therapy in certain patients has reduced the local side effects of steroids.

4.   Angle closure

The second main mechanism of elevated pressure in eyes with uveitis is acute uveitis angle closure. There are two major subset mechanisms involved:

a) Posterior synechiae formation: in both phakic and pseudophakic patients between the posterior iris surface and posterior chamber intraocular lens or anterior hyaloids face. When posterior synechiae are extensive, the trabecular outflow system is impeded accumulating fluid in the posterior chamber. This high fluid accumulation in that site may produce an iris bombé, which allow contacting the anterior iris surface and the trabecular meshwork causing acute angle closure. This event may be seen on certain types of uveitis more frequently: HLA B27 associated uveitis and granulomatous uveitis including sarcoidosis, VKH and lens induced uveitis.

b) Uveal effusion is the other mechanism responsible for the acute uveitic angle closure. This is produced by the development of an inflammatory serous choroidal detachment. As the suprachoroidal space is continuous with the supraciliary space, serous effusions can track anteriorly to cause detachment and rotation with anterior displacement of the ciliary body. If the displacement is enough, the ciliary body can push the peripheral iris root forward to produce angle closure. This process is uncommon but it has been described in VKH patients, sympathetic ophthalmia and certain scleritis [27].

c) Neovascular angle membranes can cause synechial angle closure rarely, and neovascular glaucoma may develop as in patients with retinal vascular disease or ocular ischemia [24].

CLINIC EVALUATION AND DIAGNOSIS

Appropriate management of uveitic glaucoma requires an accurate diagnosis of the uveitic entity, the mechanism of aqueous outflow obstruction, and an assessment of the damage to the optic nerve.

1. Diagnosis of the Uveitis

A useful diagnostic classification of uveitis is based on the predominant anatomic site of the inflammation as described by the International Uveitis Study Group [11]. At the same time it is important to diagnoses the etiology of the intraocular inflammatory disease, the inflammatory activity status and the course of the disease.

a) According to anatomic site of inflammation: Anatomically uveitis are divided in 4 categories: anterior uveitis, intermediate uveitis, posterior uveitis and panuveitis [11]. The differentiation among this 4 categories is important at the time of decide an appropriate management to uveitic glaucoma. Some reports establish that the IOP level is higher in anterior uveitis [12, 14]. Other authors pointed that all the cases of inflammatory glaucoma in acute and chronic uveitis were in patients with anterior segment inflammation, regardless of the primary site of inflammation [36]. However there are also authors that establish that there are no differences in the development of raised IOP in the different anatomic types of uveitis [2].

b) According to etiology of the intraocular inflammatory disease: The etiology is crucial to make an appropriate treatment of the uveitis, the absence of control of the inflammatory process conduce to an absence of control of the inflammatory glaucoma. Although there are authors who reports no differences among the different causes of uveitis [2], the most of the studies report JRA, Fuchs' cyclitis, Posner-Schlossman syndrome, and herpetic keratouveitis as the most frequent causes of uveitic glaucoma [27]. Among then one report suggests that the IOP in Possner-Schlossman syndrome is significantly higher than in all other uveitis entities [14].

c) According to the inflammatory activity status: The activity of anterior chamber inflammation should be on the basis of the cells in the anterior chamber. Inactive uveitis is defined as rare cells or less. The presence of at least one cell in every field is indicative of active uveitis. There is no consensus on a definition of inactive vitritis [11]. In a study the majority of the patients with uveitis and high IOP had significant symptoms of active inflammation. According to this study in Possner-Schlossman syndrome, herpetic uveitis and HLA-B27-related acute anterior uveitis, all eyes had active inflammation in the anterior segment of the eye when IOP was high and in Behcet disease, the majority of eyes had no active inflammation in the anterior segment of the eye when IOP increased [14].

d) According to the course of the disease: The uveitis can be classified as acute, recurrent and chronic uveitis. The term acute is used to describe the course of specific uveitic syndromes characterized by sudden onset and limited duration. The term recurrent is used to describe repeated episodes of uveitis separated by periods of inactivity without treatment, in which these periods of inactivity without treatment are at least 3 months in duration. The term chronic is used to describe persistent uveitis characterized by prompt relapse (in less than 3 months) after discontinuation of therapy. The majority of the studies point chronic uveitis as the main factor associated to uveitic glaucoma [12, 36].

2. Mechanism of Aqueous Outflow Obstruction

a) Gonioscopy. Assessment of the anterior chamber angle is critically important in determining why the IOP is elevated and developing a logical treatment strategy. Gonioscopy is essential to differentiate between an open and closed angle. With indentation gonioscopy, the presence of peripheral anterior synechiae (PAS) can be excluded in cases with appositional closure (Figure 1). Other angle features, such as trabecular meshwork pigmentation, should be documented. Gonioscopy may also reveal the cause of the IOP rise, such as retained lens cortex in the angle after catarac surgery or a microscopic silicone oil hyperoleum in the upper angle. The angle may be open or closed irrespective of the type of uveitis especially if there has been prior intraocular surgery. For example, when glaucoma presents in patients with Posner-Schlossman syndrome or Fuchs' heterochromiccyclitis the angle is typically open. Inflammatory posterior synechiae or PAS do not develop in these conditions by definition. In some patients, the resulting synechial secondary angle closure may be superimposed on chronic open-angle glaucoma secondary to intraocular inflammation or corticosteroid therapy, or even pre-existing primary open-angle glaucoma. Rarely neovascular membranes can cause synechial angle closure and neovascular glaucoma may develop. The presence of PAS and its width was evaluated in a study. In this study, 8% of the eyes had PAS wider than 180° of the trabecular meshwork, 37% with PAS smaller than 180° and 55% had no synechiaes. PAS were more frequently seen in sarcoidosis, although the majority were smaller than 180° [14].

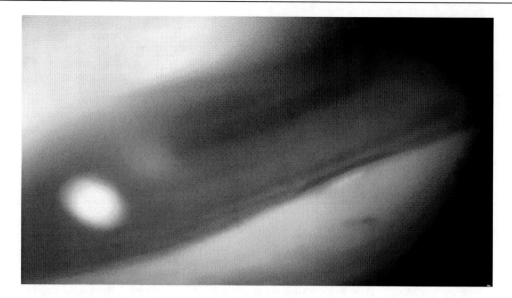

Figure 1. Presence of peripheral anterior synechiae (PAS) in gonioscopy.

3. Assessment of the Damage to the Optic Nerve.

a) Optic nerve. A proper optic nerve assessment is essential. The presence of optic nerve damage is not a prerequisite to aggressive management if the IOP is very high, although strictly speaking the diagnosis should be one of secondary ocular hypertension rather than glaucoma in the absence of optic nerve damage [10]. Baseline photographs of the optic nerve and chronologic comparisons for changes can be really useful.

b) Visual Field.When evaluating patients with an elevated IOP and uveitis, examination of the optic nerve and visual field allows the clinician to assess for glaucomatous damage. One study report that the majority of patients with raised IOP and uveitis did not have any abnormality in the visual field [14]. Even this study reports that none of the eyes with Possner-Schlossman syndrome and HLA-B27-related acute anterior uveitis had an abnormal visual field [14].

c) Others. When gonioscopy can be difficult to perform in individuals with a cloudy cornea. High-resolution ultrasound biomicroscopy (UBM, Paradigm Medical Industries Inc., Salt Lake City, UT) is useful for evaluating the anterior chamber angle and ciliary body when corneal edema obstructs the gonioscopic view. Although the clinical examination is paramount, adjunctive techniques for measuring the nerve fiber layer or optic nerve contour are helpful. The nerve fiber analyzer (GDx, Laser Diagnostic Technologies Inc., San Diego, CA), optical coherence tomography (OCT, Humphrey-Zeiss, Dublin, CA), and Heidelberg retina tomography (HRT, Heidelberg Engineering, GmbH, Dossenheim, Germany) have permitted improved and more objective evaluation of the nerve fiber layer and optic nerve.

ETIOLOGY

Increased IOP can occur in any type of ocular inflammation and may develop a subsequent glaucomatous neuropathy. Multiple etiologies have been described responsible to uveitic glaucoma (Table 1) [23]. However, there are causal agents or states more related to uveitic glaucoma due to several factors such as hypertensive character, gradual mild onset or chronic evolution among others features:

1. Herpetic Uveitis

Herpetic uveitis are caused by herpes virus infections and recognized as most important cause ofIOHS, which may result from herpes simplex virus, varicella zoster virus or cytomegalovirus.

a) Herpes simplex virus (HSV): up to one-third of patients with herpetic uveitis develop IOHS, but only 10% uveitic glaucoma [16]. A presumed diagnosis can often be done based on the presence of prior or active corneal involvement (epithelial keratitis, stromal keratitis and keratouveitis) or decreased corneal sensation. The presence of patchy or sectorial iris atrophy suggests herpetic uveitis but is not pathognomonic of this virus (Figure 2). The elevated IOP is thought caused by trabecullitis, inflammatory obstruction of trabecular meshwork [16] and angle closure in severe keratouveitis.

b) Varicella zoster virus (VZV): up to two-third of patients with VZV reactivation in the distribution of trigeminal nerve has ocular involvement and nearly half of all patients with anterior segment inflammation will develop an IOHS. Either patchy or sectorial iris atrophy may also be present. IOP elevated and glaucoma may be caused by decreased outflow facility due to trabecullar obstruction from inflammatory debris, trabecullitis and damage to trabecular meshwork by recurrent inflammation [37]. Systemic acyclovir early appears useful to reduce viral proliferation and the risk of complications such as uveitis and elevated IOP [38].

c) Cytomegalovirus (CMV): although serologic evidence of systemic CMV infection is quiet high in most population, the ocular infection typically develops in immunocompromised patients, where necrotizing retinitis is the most common ocular presentation and glaucoma can go with it. However, the association between CMV and immunocompetent patients has been recently recognized based on CMV DNA by polymerase chain reaction (PCR). Intraocular antibodies directed against CMV have been identified in the absence of HSV and VZV DNA in aqueous fluid sampled from these patients. CMV-associated anterior uveitis presents chronic or recurrent unilateral anterior chamber inflammation and elevated IOP. A specific therapeutic regimen typically with gancyclovir can be useful and used to support the diagnosis.

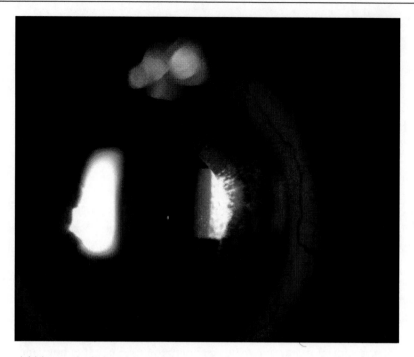

Figure 2. Sectorial iris atrophy in herpetic uveitis.

2. Fuchs' Uveitis

This condition is usually unilateral, affects adults individuals (between the third and the fifth decades) with the insidious onset of mild, chronic anterior uveitis that is usually asymptomatic. Cataract (50%) and glaucoma (14%) are the most common complications of this entity [39]. Bilateral cases are extremely rare but appear to have a higher incidence of glaucoma [40]. The risk of development of glaucoma after presentation with Fuchs' uveitis varies from 0.5% to 4% per year [41]. The cause of glaucoma is due to a reduced outflow facility associated to a breakdown of the blood-aqueous barrier increasing the IOP. Gonioscopic examination reveals an open angle with multiple fine blood vessels arranged either radially or concentrically in the trabecular meshwork. These vessels tend to bleed after puncture of the anterior chamber or minor trauma. Subtle heterochromia may be observed in the eye affected especially in patients with lighter and thicker iris.

3. GlaucomatocyclitisCrisis or Posner-SchlossmanSyndrome

This entity is characterized by recurrent episodes of mild unilateral anterior uveitis associated with elevated IOP and absence of posterior synechiae. On the other hand, the IOP during an episode is quiet high with regard to inflammation rate in the anterior chamber. Furthermore, a small number of isolated keratic precipitates are observed. The attacks last several weeks (usually up to one month) with minimal symptoms by the patients. Several agents have been postulated as responsible to this disease: HSV, VZV, CMV and rubella antibodies have been found in aqueous humor of these patients. During the attack, a reduction of outflow facility and an increased aqueous humor production are present [42]. This entity is a self-limited ocular hypertension and resolves spontaneously regardless of treatment. The differential diagnosis between Fuchs' uveitis with secondary glaucoma and the Posner-Schlossman syndrome may sometimes be difficult. Although they have some features in common, their differences can be exemplified by the dramatic response of the glaucoma in the Posner-Schlossman syndrome to a small dose of corticosteroid, whereas in Fuchs' uveitis the glaucoma does not respond so well to corticosteroids.

Therefore, an etiologic connection between these two syndromes is unlikely, although differentiating them may be difficult [41].

4. Juvenile Rheumatoid Arthritis (JRA)

It is defined as arthritis of at least three months duration that begins prior to age 16 and is diagnosed after exclusion of other causes of arthropathy [43]. It is divided in 3 subset groups depending on age of onset and, degree of articular and systemic involvement during the first 3 months: Still's disease, polyarticular and pauciarticular varieties. It affects mostly both eyes (although asymmetric) with nongranulomatouskeratic precipitates in the inferior half of the corneal endothelium. In most children the iridocyclitis is mild, insidious, chronic and asymptomatic showing posterior synechiae and pigment deposition on the anterior capsule [23]. Glaucoma is a common complication of chronic uveitis in JRA patients. The incidence of glaucoma in these patients varies from 14% to 22% and increases with the duration of the disease [43]. Steroid-induced glaucoma is also frequent because of the long-term and multiple attacks the steroids are used for controlling the inflammation. Thus, in these situations immunomodulatory treatments would be the ideal choice.

DIFFERENTIAL DIAGNOSIS

Several entities are capable of mimicking uveitis associated with a high IOP. These include Schwartz-Matsuo syndrome, pigment dispersion syndrome, microhyphema, lens-induced uveitis,nonuveitic angle closure with secondary iritis, and anterior segment ischemia.

1. Schwartz Matsuo Syndrome

The Schwartz-Matsuo syndrome is characterized by rhegmatogenous retinal detachment associated with elevated IOP (usually rhegmatogenous retinal detachment in associated with a mild reduction in IOP) and anterior uveitis [44]. It remains unclear whether the increased IOP is secondary to the anterior uveitis, concomitant damage to the trabecular meshwork, or blockage of the trabecular meshwork from retinal pigment epithelium or components of the photoreceptors [45]. Recognition of an underlying retinal detachment is essential to make the diagnosis together with careful biomicroscopic analysis of the anterior chamber cellular reaction, as the shed photoreceptors are smaller and more pigmented than leucocytes.

2. Pigment Dispersion Syndrome

Pigment dispersion syndrome, a common condition in young myopic patients, is characterized by a posterior bowing of the iris, which causes rubbing of the pigmented iris epithelium against lens structures, liberation of pigment into the anterior chamber (AC). Dispersed pigmented cells, which are often mistaken for inflammatory cells, can deposit on the anterior lens surface, on the corneal endothelium forming a Krukenberg spindle, or in the trabecular meshwork, thereby compromising aqueous outflow. Radial, spoke-like transillumination defects are often present [46]. Anterior uveitis can cause iris pigment epithelitis with the release of pigment, inflammatory cells and debris into the AC, which can be mistaken for pigment dispersion syndrome.The loss of pigment epithelial cells is often associated with iris trans-illumination defects.Herpetic uveitis is a common cause of iris transillumination defects associated with elevated IOP. Furthermore, uveitis can cause patchy increased trabecular meshwork pigmentation.

3. Microhyphema

Microhypema is a suspension of red blood cells in the AC without clot formation and is most often seen after blunt ocular trauma or previous ocular surgery. While an uncommon complication with modern intraocular lenses, microhyphema and inflammation following cataract surgery as a result of iris chafing from the edges or loops of the intraocular lens has been observed as part of the uveitis-glaucoma-hyphema syndrome. Acute ocular hypertension can develop in up to 10% of patients with microhyphema and usually results from deposition of red blood cells, platelets, or fibrin in the trabecular meshwork. IOP often normalizes as the microhyphema resolves.

4. Lens Induced Uveitis

Ocular hypertension in patients with lens-induced uveitis is believed to result from either deposition of lens material and/or lens material-laden macrophages in the trabecular meshwork [47]. Two kind of lens-induced hypertension are described:

a) Phacolytic glaucoma occurs when a hypermature cataract leaks liquefied cortical material into the anterior chamber. Macrophages are found in the aqueous humor, although keratic precipitates are rare. Treatment involves suppressing the inflammation with topical corticosteroids and removing the cataract.

b) Phacoantigenic/Phacotoxic glaucoma occurs after recent cataract extraction or traumatic rupture of the lens capsule, and is characterized by conjunctival-chemosis and anterior segment inflammation that develops within days to weeks after the capsular disruption. In these patients inflammation is treated with topical, periocular, or systemic corticosteroids in addition to antiglaucoma medications.

5. Non-Uveitic Angle Closure with Secondary Iritis

Patients with acute nonuveitic angle closure typically have mild anterior chamber inflammation that may mimic IOHS. Gonioscopy of both eyes will usually reveal narrow angles in these patients and thus allow IOHS to be excluded.

6. Anterior Segment Ischemia

Anterior segment ischemia caused by carotid artery insufficiency may simulate an anterior uveitis in older patients with the presence of cells and flare. The amount of flare is often out of proportion to the number of cells in the anterior chamber compared to other types of anterior uveitis. Usually it is accompanied by a high IOP. The pupil is poorly reactive, and patients often complain of dull, deep, and chronic pain. Anterior segment ischemia is often associated with other signs of ischemia, such as venous stasis and neovascularization. Therapy should be focused on improving the ischemia rather than treating the secondary ocular findings [48].

MANAGEMENT

When dealing with uveitic glaucoma it is essential to identify the underling mechanism of elevated IOP, thus a careful gonioscopic evaluation is compulsory.

It may be helpful to set an acceptable target IOP as in many uveitic glaucoma patients the optic nerve can be relatively spared. It is also important to determine the time and course of the IOP elevation, hypertension related to episodes may be treated with medication during the event. Exhaustive control of inflammation is extremely important as it may control undesirable secondary effects such as synechial formation, and also the surgical results are worse when surgery is performed prior to control of the intraocular inflammatory disease [49].Good control of intraocular inflammation for a minimum of 3 months before surgery is ideal but may not be practical because glaucoma surgery in uveitis is rarely performed on an elective basis. Similarly the relapse of the uveitis after the surgery is associated with a higher percentage of surgical failure [49]. So the control of the inflammatory process is crucial not only before of surgery but also after it to achieve a success.

Another important factor to have in mind is the response to corticosteroids, but long-term effects of inflammation are more severe than a short term IOP fluctuation in the case of a positive responder [27].

1. Angle Closure

Pupil block induced glaucoma is treated with Nd-Yag laser iridotomy, but if inflammation is active, this may be less successful and a surgical iridectomy may be needed. Intracameral tissue plasminogen inhibitor may be useful to treat pupil block in patients with acute fibrinous uveitis [50]. In aphakic eyes, laser iridotomy can be easily occluded by the vitreous and the surgical iridectomy is the preferred treatment if this situation happens.

Neovascular angle closure secondary to retinal ischemia is best treated with retinal photocoagulation and if peripheral anterior synechiae has not developed it may improve aqueous outflow throughout the trabecular meshwork and may avoid the need of surgery [24]. On the other hand, synechial angle closure without pupil block can be treated initially with medications but surgery is most likely to be required [27].

2. Medical Management of Increased IOP

When possible, uveitic glaucoma may be treated with topical medications, response to topical hypotensive medications may vary in uveitic glaucoma. Topical Beta-blockers are usually the first line of therapy, but in some patients its effect can be weak [27]. Metipranolol, which is rarely used nowadays, has been associated with anterior granulomatous uveitis and should be avoided [51]. According to the IOP level the second line of treatment may be a systemic Carbonic Anhydrase Inhibitor (CAI) as acetazolamide. However, if IOP levels are not extremely elevated, topical CAIs or alpha-adrenergic agonists may be considered. Anterior uveitis associated with brimonidine use has been reported and brimonidine should be used with caution or avoided if possible [52].

Prostaglandin analogues are potent topical medications and are not associated with increased risk of cystoid macular edema or anterior uveitis [53]however,latanoprost must be used with caution or avoided if possible when there is a history of herpetic disease as it may precipitate recurrences [54].

3. Surgical Management

If good IOP control is not achieved with medications and optic nerve damage is present, surgery must be considered. However, chronic uveitic glaucoma carries a high risk of surgical failure in the long term and may require more post-operative therapeutic interventions to control the IOP [55].

The use of antifibrotic agents is a common practice when dealing with these patients. Hypotony is a high risk in uveitic glaucoma as if in the post-operative period aqueous humour production decreases, any filtration might be excessive and hypotony may develop. This condition may be avoided with a tight scleral flap closure [27].

Phacotrabeculectomy associated with Mitomycin C is a safe and effective option when a secondary cataract coexists with uveitic glaucoma, if an adequate suppression of the inflammation is reached [56] (Figure 3). However, there are studies reporting that trabeculectomy alone is better than the combined surgeries [57]. In a study of our group it was found worse results with the combined surgery than with trabeculectomy alone, which seems to cause less post-operative flare than cataract surgery in isolation [58], possibly explaining the better success of trabeculectomy alone in primary open angle glaucoma than the combined surgery [59]. It is likely that this effect is exaggerated in uveitis, and the combined cataract and glaucoma surgery may not be appropriate. Although some studies reported good outcomes combined phacoemulsification approaches in uveitic glaucoma [56], however there is not prospective studies which compares the success rate for combined phacoemulsification and trabeculectomy approaches in uveitic glaucoma, so further studies are warranted.

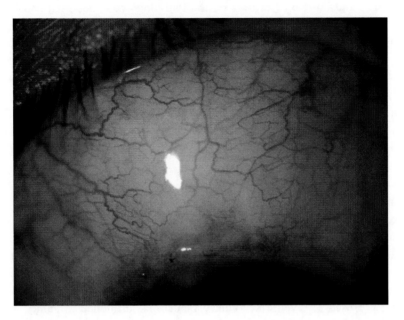

Figure 3. Phacotrabeculectomy associated with Mitomycin C in uveitic glaucoma 1 day post-surgery.

Glaucoma drainage devices (GDD) have been used with increasing frequency. Molteno reported the best results for GDD implantation with a long-term follow-up with 87% achieving an IOP between 5–21 mmHg on 0.41 medications [60]. Another study with the Baerveldt GDD obtained a success rate of 91.7% at 24 months [61]. Also there are reports suggesting Ahmed valve as the first option in uveitic glaucoma [62, 63].

The new approaches such as deep sclerectomy have been also applied in the case of uveitic glaucoma without significative differences with traditional trabeculectomy [64].

Cyclodestructive procedures must be used with extreme caution in patients with uveitis, as it may exacerbate inflammation and may also precipitate phthisis and should be reserved for patients with refractory glaucoma secondary to chronic mild inflammatory disease [65].

REFERENCES

[1]   Durrani OM, Tehrani NN, Marr JE, Moradi P, Stavrou P, Murray PI. Degree, duration, and causes of visual loss in uveitis. *Br. J.Ophthalmol.* Sep 2004;88(9):1159-1162.

[2]   Neri P, Azuara-Blanco A, Forrester JV. Incidence of glaucoma in patients with uveitis. *J. Glaucoma.* Dec 2004;13(6):461-465.

[3]   Beer   GJ.   *Lehre   von   den   Augenkrankheiten :alsLeitfadenzuseinenöffentlichenVorlesungenentworfen.* Wien: Camesina :Heubner und Volke; 1813.

[4]   Hischberg J. *The History of Ophthalmology.*Vol 6. Bonn: JP Wayenburgh; 1985.

[5]   vonGraefe A. Über die IridectomiebeiGlaucom und über den glaucomatösen Process. *Arch.Für.Ophthalmologie.* 1857;3:456-560.

[6]   Weber A. Die Ursache des Glaucoms. *Arch. Für.Ophthalmologie.* 1877;23:1-91.

[7]   Smith P. Erasmus Wilson Lectures on the Pathology of Glaucoma. *Br. Med. J.* Apr 13 1889;1(1476):817-824.

[8]   Fuchs E. Ueberkomplikationen der heterochromie. *Z Augenheilkd.* 1906;15:191-212.

[9]   Posner A, Schlossman A. Syndrome of glaucomato-cyclitic crises. *Am. J.Ophthalmol.* Jun 1948;31(6):735.

[10]   Foster PJ, Buhrmann R, Quigley HA, Johnson GJ. The definition and classification of glaucoma in prevalence surveys. *Br. J.Ophthalmol.* Feb 2002;86(2):238-242.

[11]   Jabs DA, Nussenblatt RB, Rosenbaum JT. Standardization of uveitis nomenclature for reporting clinical data. Results of the First International Workshop. *Am. J.Ophthalmol.* Sep 2005;140(3):509-516.

[12]   Merayo-Lloves J, Power WJ, Rodriguez A, Pedroza-Seres M, Foster CS. Secondary glaucoma in patients with uveitis. *Ophthalmologica.* 1999;213(5):300-304.

[13]   Herbert HM, Viswanathan A, Jackson H, Lightman SL. Risk factors for elevated intraocular pressure in uveitis. *J. Glaucoma.* Apr 2004;13(2):96-99.

[14]   Takahashi T, Ohtani S, Miyata K, Miyata N, Shirato S, Mochizuki M. A clinical evaluation of uveitis-associated secondary glaucoma. *Jpn J.Ophthalmol.* Sep-Oct 2002;46(5):556-562.

[15]   Ascaso FJ, Bosch J. Uveitic secondary glaucoma: influence in James Joyce's (1882-1941) last works. *J Med Biogr.* Feb 2010;18(1):57-60.

[16]   Falcon MG, Williams HP. Herpes simplex kerato-uveitis and glaucoma. *Trans OphthalmolSoc U K.* Apr 1978;98(1):101-104.

[17]   Jabs DA, Johns CJ. Ocular involvement in chronic sarcoidosis. *Am. J.Ophthalmol.* Sep 15 1986;102(3):297-301.

[18]   Westfall AC, Lauer AK, Suhler EB, Rosenbaum JT. Toxoplasmosis retinochoroiditis and elevated intraocular pressure: a retrospective study. *J. Glaucoma.* Feb 2005;14(1):3-10.

[19]   Reddy S, Cubillan LD, Hovakimyan A, Cunningham ET, Jr. Inflammatory ocular hypertension syndrome (IOHS) in patients with syphilitic uveitis. *Br. J.Ophthalmol.* Dec 2007;91(12):1610-1612.

[20]   Clark AF. Basic sciences in clinical glaucoma: steroids, ocular hypertension, and glaucoma. *J. Glaucoma.* Oct 1995;4(5):354-369.

[21]   Jones R, 3rd, Rhee DJ. Corticosteroid-induced ocular hypertension and glaucoma: a brief review and update of the literature. *Curr. Opin.Ophthalmol.* Apr 2006;17(2):163-167.

[22]   Goldstein DA, Godfrey DG, Hall A, et al. Intraocular pressure in patients with uveitis treated with fluocinoloneacetonide implants. *Arch.Ophthalmol.* Nov 2007;125(11):1478-1485.

[23]   Moorthy RS, Mermoud A, Baerveldt G, Minckler DS, Lee PP, Rao NA. Glaucoma associated with uveitis. *Surv. Ophthalmol.* Mar-Apr 1997;41(5):361-394.

[24]   Kuchtey RW, Lowder CY, Smith SD. Glaucoma in patients with ocular inflammatory disease. *OphthalmolClin North Am.* Sep 2005;18(3):421-430, vii.

[25]   Grant WM. Clinical measurements of aqueous outflow. *AMA Arch.Ophthalmol.* Aug 1951;46(2):113-131.

[26]   Barsotti MF, Bartels SP, Freddo TF, Kamm RD. The source of protein in the aqueous humor of the normal monkey eye. *Invest.Ophthalmol. Vis. Sci.* Mar 1992;33(3):581-595.

[27]   Kok H, Barton K. Uveitic glaucoma. *Ophthalmol.Clin. North Am.* Sep 2002;15(3):375-387, viii.

[28]   Edelsten C, Lee V, Bentley CR, Kanski JJ, Graham EM. An evaluation of baseline risk factors predicting severity in juvenile idiopathic arthritis associated uveitis and other chronic anterior uveitis in early childhood. *Br. J.Ophthalmol.* Jan 2002;86(1):51-56.

[29]   Kotaniemi K, Sihto-Kauppi K. Occurrence and management of ocular hypertension and secondary glaucoma in juvenile idiopathic arthritis-associated uveitis: An observational series of 104 patients. *Clin.Ophthalmol.* Dec 2007;1(4):455-459.

[30]   Alvarado JA, Murphy CG. Outflow obstruction in pigmentary and primary open angle glaucoma. *Arch.Ophthalmol.* Dec 1992;110(12):1769-1778.

[31]   Becker B. Intraocular Pressure Response to Topical Corticosteroids. *Invest.Ophthalmol.* Apr 1965;4:198-205.

[32]   Wilson K, McCartney MD, Miggans ST, Clark AF. Dexamethasone induced ultrastructural changes in cultured human trabecular meshwork cells. *Curr. Eye Res.* Sep 1993;12(9):783-793.

[33]   Clark AF, Lane D, Wilson K, Miggans ST, McCartney MD. Inhibition of dexamethasone-induced cytoskeletal changes in cultured human trabecular meshwork cells by tetrahydrocortisol. *Invest.Ophthalmol. Vis. Sci.* Apr 1996;37(5):805-813.

[34]   Steely HT, Browder SL, Julian MB, Miggans ST, Wilson KL, Clark AF. The effects of dexamethasone on fibronectin expression in cultured human trabecular meshwork cells. *Invest.Ophthalmol. Vis Sci.* Jun 1992;33(7):2242-2250.

[35]   Snyder RW, Stamer WD, Kramer TR, Seftor RE. Corticosteroid treatment and trabecular meshwork proteases in cell and organ culture supernatants. *Exp. Eye Res.* Oct 1993;57(4):461-468.

[36]   Panek WC, Holland GN, Lee DA, Christensen RE. Glaucoma in patients with uveitis. *Br. J.Ophthalmol.* Apr 1990;74(4):223-227.

[37]   Hedges TR, 3rd, Albert DM. The progression of the ocular abnormalities of herpes zoster. Histopathologic observations of nine cases. *Ophthalmology.* Feb 1982;89(2):165-177.

[38]   Cobo LM, Foulks GN, Liesegang T, et al. Oral acyclovir in the therapy of acute herpes zoster ophthalmicus. An interim report. *Ophthalmology.* Nov 1985;92(11):1574-1583.

[39]   Alanko HI, Vuorre I, Saari KM. Characteristics of corneal endothelial cells in Fuchs' heterochromiccyclitis. *ActaOphthalmol. (Copenh).* Dec 1986;64(6):623-631.

[40]   Huber A. [Glaucoma in complicated heterochromia of Fuchs]. *Ophthalmologica.* Feb 1961;141:122-135.

[41]   Jones NP. Glaucoma in Fuchs' Heterochromic Uveitis: aetiology, management and outcome. *Eye (Lond).* 1991;5 (Pt 6):662-667.

[42]   Spivey BE, Armaly MF. Tonographic findings in glaucomatocyclitic crises. *Am. J.Ophthalmol.* Jan 1963;55:47-51.

[43]   Calabro JJ, Parrino GR, Atchoo PD, Marchesano JM, Goldberg LS. Chronic iridocyclitis in juvenile rheumatoid arthritis. *Arthritis Rheum.* Jul-Aug 1970;13(4):406-413.

[44] Schwartz A. Chronic open-angle glaucoma secondary to rhegmatogenous retinal detachment. *Am. J.Ophthalmol.* Feb 1973;75(2):205-211.

[45] Matsuo T. Photoreceptor outer segments in aqueous humor: key to understanding a new syndrome. *Surv. Ophthalmol.* Nov-Dec 1994;39(3):211-233.

[46] Niyadurupola N, Broadway DC. Pigment dispersion syndrome and pigmentary glaucoma--a major review. *Clin. Experiment.Ophthalmol.* Dec 2008;36(9):868-882.

[47] Irvine SR, Irvine AR, Jr. Lens-induced uveitis and glaucoma. II. The "phacotoxic" reaction. *Am. J.Ophthalmol.* Mar 1952;35(3):370-375; contd.

[48] Mendrinos E, Machinis TG, Pournaras CJ. Ocular ischemic syndrome. *Surv. Ophthalmol.* Jan-Feb 2010;55(1):2-34.

[49] Carreno E, Villarón S, Portero A, Herreras JM, Maquet JA, Calonge M. Surgical outcomes of uveitic glaucoma. *Journal of Ophthalmic Inflammation and Infection.* 2010.

[50] Skolnick CA, Fiscella RG, Tessler HH, Goldstein DA. Tissue plasminogen activator to treat impending pupillary block glaucoma in patients with acute fibrinous HLA-B27 positive iridocyclitis. *Am. J.Ophthalmol.* Mar 2000;129(3):363-366.

[51] O'Connor GR. Granulomatous uveitis and metipranolol. *Br. J.Ophthalmol.* Aug 1993;77(8):536-538.

[52] Byles DB, Frith P, Salmon JF. Anterior uveitis as a side effect of topical brimonidine. *Am. J.Ophthalmol.* Sep 2000;130(3):287-291.

[53] Chang JH, McCluskey P, Missotten T, Ferrante P, Jalaludin B, Lightman S. Use of ocular hypotensive prostaglandin analogues in patients with uveitis: does their use increase anterior uveitis and cystoid macular oedema? *Br. J.Ophthalmol.* Jul 2008;92(7):916-921.

[54] Wand M, Gilbert CM, Liesegang TJ. Latanoprost and herpes simplex keratitis. *Am. J.Ophthalmol.* May 1999;127(5):602-604.

[55] Noble J, Derzko-Dzulynsky L, Rabinovitch T, Birt C. Outcome of trabeculectomy with intraoperative mitomycin C for uveitic glaucoma. *Can. J.Ophthalmol.* Feb 2007;42(1):89-94.

[56] Park UC, Ahn JK, Park KH, Yu HG. Phacotrabeculectomy with mitomycin C in patients with uveitis. *Am. J.Ophthalmol.* Dec 2006;142(6):1005-1012.

[57] Murthy SK, Damji KF, Pan Y, Hodge WG. Trabeculectomy and phacotrabeculectomy, with mitomycin-C, show similar two-year target IOP outcomes. *Can. J.Ophthalmol.* Feb 2006;41(1):51-59.

[58] Siriwardena D, Kotecha A, Minassian D, Dart JK, Khaw PT. Anterior chamber flare after trabeculectomy and after phacoemulsification. *Br. J.Ophthalmol.* Sep 2000;84(9):1056-1057.

[59] Park HJ, Weitzman M, Caprioli J. Temporal corneal phacoemulsification combined with superior trabeculectomy. A retrospective case-control study. *Arch.Ophthalmol.* Mar 1997;115(3):318-323.

[60] Molteno AC, Whittaker KW, Bevin TH, Herbison P. Otago Glaucoma Surgery Outcome Study: long term results of cataract extraction combined with Molteno implant insertion or trabeculectomy in primary glaucoma. *Br. J.Ophthalmol.* Jan 2004;88(1):32-35.

[61] Ceballos EM, Parrish RK, 2nd, Schiffman JC. Outcome of Baerveldt glaucoma drainage implants for the treatment of uveitic glaucoma. *Ophthalmology.* Dec 2002;109(12):2256-2260.

[62] Rachmiel R, Trope GE, Buys YM, Flanagan JG, Chipman ML. Ahmed glaucoma valve implantation in uveitic glaucoma versus open-angle glaucoma patients. *Can. J.Ophthalmol.* Aug 2008;43(4):462-467.

[63] Papadaki TG, Zacharopoulos IP, Pasquale LR, Christen WB, Netland PA, Foster CS. Long-term results of Ahmed glaucoma valve implantation for uveitic glaucoma. *Am. J.Ophthalmol.* Jul 2007;144(1):62-69.

[64] Dupas B, Fardeau C, Cassoux N, Bodaghi B, LeHoang P. Deep sclerectomy and trabeculectomy in uveitic glaucoma. *Eye (Lond).* Feb 2010;24(2):310-314.

[65] Schlote T, Derse M, Zierhut M. Transscleral diode laser cyclophotocoagulation for the treatment of refractory glaucoma secondary to inflammatory eye diseases. *Br. J.Ophthalmol.* Sep 2000;84(9):999-1003.

In: Glaucoma: Etiology, Pathogenesis and Treatments
Editors: Z. G. Fei and S. Zeng

ISBN: 978-1-61470-975-6
© 2012 Nova Science Publishers, Inc.

Chapter V

Selective Laser Trabeculoplasty: A Promising Treatment for Open Angle Glaucoma

*Eman Elhawy[1], Gautam Kamthan[2] and John Danias[1]**

[1]Department of Ophthalmology, SUNY Downstate Medical School, Brooklyn, NY,
[2]Department of Ophthalmology, Mount Sinai Medical School, New York, NY

ABSTRACT

Selective laser trabeculoplasty (SLT) is a therapeutic modality that utilizes Neodymium: Yttrium aluminium garnet (Nd:YAG) laser to increase outflow facility in the trabecular meshwork(TM). It selectively targets pigmented cells in the trabecular meshwork causing little if any damage to trabecular cells. It presumably increases outflow facility by altering the composition of the extracellular matrix of the TM.

SLT efficacy, safety, and repeatability have been extensively studied. SLT is equally effective to Argon Laser Trabeculoplasty (ALT) achieving on average a 20% reduction on intraocular pressure (IOP) despite causing significantly less histologic damage to TM. However, similarly to ALT SLT loses effectiveness over time and is occasionally accompanied by IOP spikes immediately after the procedure.

SLT is effective irrespective of the amount of TM pigmentation and is particularly effective in secondary open angle glaucomas including pseudoexfoliation and pigmentary glaucoma. The only variable predictive of SLT success is IOP before the procedure.

The major theoretical advantage of SLT over ALT is its potential for virtually limitless repeatability. However this advantage remains largely theoretical as there are few studies proving the efficacy of such repeatability.

SLT is promising as single therapeutic intervention in third world countries because of the low rate of complications, the ease of application and the potential for repeat therapy. Although economic modeling has been used to advocate for widespread use in managed care environments, the economic advantages from a public health perspective in this setting are questionable.

* Corresponding author: John Danias, MD, PhD SUNY Downstate Medical Center 450 Clarkson Ave Brooklyn NY 11203 Phone: 718 270-4242 Fax: 718 270-7678 Email: John.danias@downstate.edu

Keywords: Selective laser trabeculoplasty, SLT, laser trabeculoplasty

INTRODUCTION

In 1995, Latina et al demonstrated selective damage to pigmented cells using a Neodymium: Yttrium Aluminum Garnet (Nd:YAG) laser in vitro [1]. A few years later, a multicenter study was completed showing that using this laser to treat the trabecular meshwork (TM) reduced intraocular pressure (IOP) in patients with glaucoma [2]. This treatment method came to be known as Selective Laser Trabeculoplasty (SLT).

Proponents of SLT touted it as the replacement for Argon Laser Trabeculoplasty (ALT), while others questioned whether it offers any advantage over ALT. SLT generated this debate because of its ability to reduce IOP and cause less damage than ALT to the TM. This attribute has been the basis for theories claiming that SLT could be limitlessly repeatable in the treatment of glaucoma. As SLT has been approved by the FDA for the past 10 years it is time to perform an honest appraisal of its capabilities and limitations. This chapter endeavors to explore our current knowledge about this procedure, and examine whether its attributes make SLT likely to completely replace ALT as a therapeutic option in the management of glaucoma.

HISTORY

Laser application to the TM to achieve IOP reduction was pioneered by Krasnov [3]. In 1972 he introduced the concept of direct goniopuncture using a Q-switched ruby laser. The effect, though favorable, was short lived lasting only for six months. Despite changes in duration, intensity and laser type, results remained similar. Thus goniopuncture was abandoned for trabeculoplasty using an argon laser (ALT) [4].

At a time when glaucoma management depended on the use of timolol, pilocarpine, epinephrine and oral carbonic anhydrase inhibitors, the addition of another office based surgery to the armamentarium of ophthalmologists was welcomed. A number of small studies reinforced the original reports of success using ALT [5-9].

With these findings, ALT use quickly spread. In 1990 when the Glaucoma Laser Trial (GLT) [10] showed that ALT was at least as effective as contemporary medical therapy with timolol maleate 0.5% for up to at least seven years, there was even greater confidence to employ the technique. Since then, there has been continued experience affirming ALT's safety and efficacy. While the GLT was underway, work in the lab was leading to the development of SLT. First, Anderson and Parrish [11] demonstrated that pigmented structures could be selectively damaged by applying a brief pulse of radiation that is preferentially absorbed by the pigmented cells and not the surrounding structures. Then, Latina and Park[1] showed that a Q-switched, Nd:YAG laser could cause selective death of only pigmented structures and cells in a mixed, pigmented and non pigmented, bovine trabecular meshwork cell culture . Latina and Park used the principles of selective thermolysis in their cell cultures to target pigmented structures. It was possible to confine the energy to these cells without affecting surrounding structures or causing any heat damage [1]. SLT efficacy and safety was examined on patients with uncontrolled open angle glaucoma on maximum medical therapy or previously treated with ALT and it was proven to be effective and safe [1]. SLT gained FDA approval for human use in March 2001.

MECHANISM OF ACTION

More than 30 years after the introduction of ALT the IOP lowering effect after laser application to the TM is not well understood. There are two main theories attempting to explain this effect:

1. The mechanical theory postulates that after laser application, a scar forms in the TM. This scar contracts causing traction and opening of intertrabecular spaces and Schlemm's canal and that leads to increased aqueous outflow [12]. In human and animal studies, absence of vacuoles in the inner layer of Schlemm's canal was noted beneath the laser application area suggesting no aqueous flow at this area. In addition, increased herniation of juxtacanalicular TM into Sclemm's canal was noted in the non-lasered TM. An increase in the number of vacuoles in inner Sclemm's canal in this region suggested increased aqueous outflow [13]. Although this theory may be applicable to ALT where extensive damage to the TM leads to scar formation, it is also possible that it may only be applicable to eyes with very high IOP [14].

2. The biologic theory of laser induced IOP lowering, suggests that biological effects are being induced by laser application [15]. Anterior trabecular cells are stimulated to divide in both treated and non treated areas of the TM after laser application [16]. It is presumed that these cells are multipotent cells and differentiate into TM cells and phagocytic cells that are responsible for extracellular matrix formation and clearing. Phagocytic cells clearing of the debris may result in increased outflow [17]. Laser application also induces the production of cytokines, chemotactic and vasoactive factors. Cytokines stimulate metalloprotinases expression and thus increase extracellular matrix remodeling [18] and transendothelial flow in Sclemm's canal [19]. Increase of peroxidase levels was detected in rabbit eyes following SLT and this suggests a role for oxygen free radicals in post SLT inflammation [20]. This inflammatory response including macrophage recruitment to the TM may have an important role in IOP lowering following both ALT and SLT application [12].

HISTOLOGICAL EFFECTS

The original in vitro studies by Latina and Park[1] found that SLT caused rupturing and fracturing of the lysosomal membranes and melanin granules of pigmented cells, while the non-pigmented cells were devoid of any ultrastructural damage. Findings from these studies stimulated others to compare the difference in the amount of tissue damage between SLT and ALT. Studies, using scanning and transmission electron microscopy, examined the trabecular meshwork of autopsy specimens after receiving either ALT or SLT [21]. ALT was noted to cause drastic changes to the TM: 70μm diameter cavities were found with coagulative damage along the edges and at the base and TM endothelial cells that were separating from trabecular beams, which had fragmented and lodged into trabecular spaces. Whereas ALT's damage was readily apparent, the trabecular meshwork after SLT exhibited only occasional vacuolated cells within the pigmented TM endothelium; rare pseudo-fractures of the trabecular beams; and virtually no coagulative damage. Only the pigmented cells contained damaged pigment granules. Although other investigators didn't detect such a dramatic difference in damage [12], it was apparent that ALT caused more damage than SLT especially to collagen beams as seen on electron microscopy.

SLT's sparing of the trabecular meshwork's structure can be partly explained by the lower energy delivered to the tissue. The SLT laser sends pulses of 0.8 to 1.2 mJ/pulse over a wide area with a spot diameter of 400μm. This means that 0.64-0.95 J/cm^2 are delivered with each laser application. ALT utilizes 400-800 mJ/pulse over a 50μm diameter spot which delivers 2,040-4,080 J/cm^2 per spot. The difference in damage is also due to the duration of each of the pulses [12]. An SLT pulse is applied in the order of nanoseconds compared to ALT's pulse of 0.1 seconds. Such differences can produce vastly different results. Thermal damage is confined to the target cells only if the duration of energy application is less than the thermal relaxation time. When this occurs the molecules that absorb light do not have enough time to convert the energy into heat. For melanin, thermal relaxation time is approximately 1 millisecond, so using nanosecond duration pulses as in SLT prevents thermal dissipation to surrounding structures [1]. In contrast during ALT, energy is applied over 0.1 seconds which is longer than the melanin thermal relaxation time. This long duration of laser application explains the dissipation of energy and thus the collateral damage to surrounding structures [15, 17]. Once the temperature in the tissues increases by more than 10°C, proteins begin to denature and coagulation occurs followed by necrosis that leads to scarring. This degree of damage was found to be widespread with ALT and it included Schlemm's canal and the scleral stroma [22]. Thus while ALT uses high energy, relatively long duration laser to a small area and mechanically damages the TM, SLT uses laser with much lower fluence (energy/area) [12] and of very short duration causing selective microscopic damage to pigmented cells within the TM. That is because melanin has higher energy absorption than other molecules for the wavelength (532nm) used. Thus, although SLT is applied to a much larger area selectivity of the laser used decreases histological damage to a minimum.

SAFETY

Various trials and years of experience have established that ALT is a relatively safe procedure [23]. Although experience with SLT is more limited, a number of trials have proven its high level of safety. In studies of SLT without a comparison group SLT has been found to have a safety profile comparable to that of ALT [24]. There have also been head-to-head studies comparing SLT to ALT [22, 25, 26]. The greatest concerns with SLT (similar to those experienced with ALT) are post-operative IOP spikes, intra-operative and post-operative pain, inflammation, and peripheral anterior synechiae formation.

In one study [27] 83% of eyes treated with SLT had mild to moderate inflammation within 1 hour of treatment. Inflammation decreased in 24 hours and had completely resolved in all eyes 5 days after the procedure. Pain, discomfort and blurring of vision occurred in 15% of eyes, while redness was only reported 9% of the time. Interestingly, in a study comparing SLT with ALT [28], a significant difference in post-operative pain was detected during the first 24 h after surgery with SLT inducing less pain. This difference disappeared within twenty-four hours though [28].

A major concern with ALT is the "IOP spike", a sudden rise of IOP within the first 24 h after the procedure. 25% of patients undergoing SLT had spikes of 5 mm Hg or more and 9% had a pressure elevation of greater than 8mmHg. None of the patients, however, experienced enduring elevated IOP after being treated with antiglaucoma medications [27].

The GLT [10] has previously reported that 30% of patients undergoing ALT had IOP spikes of greater than 5 mm Hg, indicating that in this respect SLT is comparable to ALT [10] although it may not be entirely appropriate to compare the results of these studies as they are vastly different in design. In trials comparing SLT with ALT directly, it was found that "IOP spikes" greater than 5 mm Hg occur in approximately 10% of patients undergoing SLT treatment versus 34% after 180 degree application of ALT [29, 30]. The amount of IOP elevation does not seem to differ between the two groups and IOP spikes usually resolve within twenty-four hours using medical treatment [27].

Other concerns with trabeculoplasty are peripheral anterior synechiae formation, retreatment rates and need for additional medical or surgical interventions. Occurrences of these complications and severity was comparable between ALT and SLT [27].

Despite SLT's general safety, severe side effects have been reported. These events emphasize the fact that SLT (as any other procedure) should only be applied after proper patient selection and appropriate informed consent. These side effects could be either a common side effect at a much higher level (like patients experiencing severe pain or patients with excessive IOP elevation) or rare adverse effects such as the occurrence of hyphema or corneal edema. Harasymowycz [31] noted that four patients with heavy pigmentation of the trabecular meshwork experienced large IOP rises (increasing by 8 to 28 mm Hg). Three patients later required trabeculectomy as a result. Hyphema occurs after SLT in some cases [32] and severe iritis and choroidal effusion have also been reported [33]. Although very rare the occurrence of severe corneal edema and haze after SLT has also been reported [34]. Anecdotal reports of induced hyperopic changes and permanent corneal haze have also been discussed among glaucoma specialists. Although not yet understood, the mechanism by which these exceedingly rare events occur may relate to pre-existing conditions in the eyes treated. Notwithstanding these isolated cases, SLT is still overall comparable in safety to ALT.

EFFICACY

It is evident from a number of studies that SLT does possess significant IOP lowering properties. In a prospective study of SLT's efficacy for long-term IOP reduction [35], using Kaplan-Meier survival analysis success rates of 60%, 53%, 44% and 44% for years 1, 2 3 and 4 after laser application were observed. Successful treatment at the time of the final follow up was defined as IOP decline by at least 3 mm Hg compared to the original IOP before treatment, keeping IOP less than or equal to 19mmHg without the need of repeated treatment together with stable field and optic nerve appearance. [35] An average decrease of 6 mm Hg (24.3% and 29.3%) was detected at 1 and 4 years, respectively.

In trials directly comparing SLT to ALT, it appears that efficacy of the former is at least as great as that of ALT's. Using ALT as a benchmark is useful because its efficacy has been firmly established following the GLT's findings [10]. In GLT [10], it was already noted that 70% of patients required further intervention after 24 months of medical therapy, whereas 56% of patients receiving ALT required intervention within the same time period. Although the GLT has since been criticized because it did not control for the effects of timolol to the contralateral eye, it did maintain a rigid treatment regimen [36] allowing establishment of ALT's efficacy.

A number of trials comparing SLT against ALT largely affirm their equivalence in terms of efficacy in lowering IOP. For example, Martinez-de-la-Casa et al [28] in a prospective study of 40 consecutive patients, divided equally between receiving ALT or SLT detected a mean percentage decrease of 22.2% for the SLT group at 6 months and 19.5% for the ALT group. These values included non-responders. Excluding non-responders, the mean percentage decrease was 26.7% for the SLT group and 21.8% for the ALT group. The differences were not statistically significant ($p=0.231$). The percentage of responders for the SLT group was 80% (16 of 20 patients) and 85% for the ALT group (17 of 20 patients), with response defined as a decrease in IOP of 3 or more mm Hg [28]. Other groups have demonstrated similar findings [27].

The above trials attempted to determine SLT efficacy in a standard comparison of two groups receiving either ALT or SLT. Others [37] have examined the efficacy of SLT in the same group of patients in order to minimize intergroup variation. These studies applied ALT to one and SLT to the other eye of the study patients. While such studies cannot control for potential contralateral effects, they also concluded that there is no statistically significant difference in IOP lowering effectiveness of SLT and ALT. Even when patients were permitted to remain on other medical therapies during follow up, results didn't differ. This lack of difference between ALT and SLT has now been extended to 5 years [22].

The single most predictive factor for SLT efficacy in terms of IOP lowering is the pre-operative IOP [38]. It was also noted that the maximum IOP ever recorded for the patient is inversely related to the SLT efficacy. Age, sex, angle pigmentation, diagnosis, or washout from previous medication do not seem to affect the IOP lowering effect of SLT [38].

REPEATABILITY

The most exciting prospect for SLT is its potential for repeatability. Based on the findings of minimal structural change to the TM caused by SLT, it has been hypothesized that there may be no limit to how many times it can be successfully applied. If this was true, one could envision managing glaucoma simply with periodic SLT application. Until recently, there was little data to support this hypothesis as most studies have not been able to recruit large enough numbers of patients that had received more than one or two sessions of SLT.

From available data, it appears that a second SLT can prove to be successful in both Caucasians and African American patients [39, 40]. Success rates of 3rd SLT are harder to determine. Every seemingly possible outcome has been reported. For example, Lai and

Bournias [41] studied second and third SLT and found that, while second SLT was beneficial, no success was achieved with a third treatment. Leon et al [39], on the other hand, found remarkable success in their third treatments. A third study by Basile and colleagues [42] examined a third and fourth SLT. Unlike the previous two studies supporting either outright success or failure, Basile and colleagues recorded mixed success with the third SLT and little to no success with a fourth SLT. This type of variability in third SLT success is likely due to the small number of patients treated in each trial (each had less than ten patients for a third SLT). Given this kind of variability, and until a larger cohort of patients is studied, it would seem that SLT can tentatively be considered to be at least partially successful when applied for the third time. Data on fourth application are rather thin at this time.

It is important to note that the term "repeatability" is used to suggest different concepts across some of the above studies. Some regard repeatability to mean specifically that a previously treated section of TM is treated again [43]. Others, such as Gulati and Latina [44], use the term "repeatability" even when SLT is applied to previously untreated sections of TM. This difference in semantics can lead to ambiguity over the true potential of SLT's "repeatability," and requires further refinement before determining the true limit of SLT repeatability.

ECONOMICS

Apart from safety and efficacy another concern with SLT is its cost. Lee and Hutnik published an important evaluation of the cost of SLT compared to single, double, or triple drug therapy [43]. This article sought to explore the potential for reducing the financial burden of multi-drug glaucoma therapy using repeat SLT treatments instead. A large number of assumptions were made, since, as discussed above, there is limited data especially on repeatability of the procedure. In addition the cost of equipment acquisition and maintenance; the cost of surgery for patients who failed treatment or had complications; and the cost of medications for patients who would require them in addition to SLT were not included in the analysis. Nonetheless, this study provides an interesting and necessary analysis of the cost-effectiveness of adopting a new technology. If SLT were repeated every two years and was equally effective to medical therapy it would save $206.54, $1668.64, $2992.67 per patient for single, double, and triple drug therapy, respectively. If SLT was repeated at three year intervals, $580.52, $2042.82, and $3366.65 could be saved per patient versus single, double, or triple drug therapy, respectively. Thus, a modest savings is possible, if all of the assumptions hold and certain costs are excluded. In an editorial [45] accompanying the above paper it is noted that, at best, and according to published data 1.5 medications on average can be replaced by SLT [45]. Based on this fact, as well as the possibility that some of the assumptions may not hold, it would be improbable for SLT to be actually cost-effective. SLT's cost-effectiveness may not, however, be an issue if it can be repeated at least twice more than ALT.

Due to the chronic nature of glaucoma the lack of trained professionals and the lifelong cost of the disease treatment, managing glaucoma patients in underdeveloped countries is particularly challenging. This is compounded by the fact that glaucoma prevalence is in many of these countries very high [46]. In these situations, where even generic medications may not be affordable and where incisional surgery may not be available because of lack of physicians, SLT performed on a periodic basis by visiting physicians or even trained members of the public may be a cost-effective alternative. Such an approach is currently being explored in St Lucia [47].

CONCLUSION

In summary since its FDA approval in 2001, SLT has become an attractive treatment option for open angle glaucoma patients. It has comparable efficacy to ALT together with high selectivity, lack of scar formation and the potential for repeatability. Although it will not necessarily completely replace ALT in the developed world, it does offer specific advantages that make it potentially appealing as a first line therapy in underdeveloped countries. The big unresolved questions are how many times SLT can be repeated and what are the chances of success of multiple SLT re-treatments.

REFERENCES

[1]   Latina, M.A. and Park, C., Selective targeting of trabecular meshwork cells: in vitro studies of pulsed and CW laser interactions. *Exp. Eye Res*, 1995; 60: 359-71.

[2]   Latina, M.A., Sibayan, S.A., Shin, D.H., Noecker, R.J., and Marcellino, G., Q-switched 532-nm Nd:YAG laser trabeculoplasty (selective laser trabeculoplasty): a multicenter, pilot, clinical study. *Ophthalmology*, 1998; 105: 2082-8; discussion 2089-90.

[3]   Krasnov, M.M., [Laser puncture of the anterior chamber angle in glaucoma (a preliminary report)]. *Vestn Oftalmol*, 1972; 3: 27-31.

[4]   Wise, J.B. and Witter, S.L., Argon laser therapy for open-angle glaucoma. A pilot study. *Arch. Ophthalmol.*, 1979; 97: 319-22.

[5]   Moulin, F. and Haut, J., [Results of argon laser treatment of 100 eyes with open-angle glaucoma (trabeculoplasty, trabeculoretraction)]. *J. Fr. Ophtalmol.*, 1983; 6: 661-70.

[6]   Spaeth, G.L., Fellman, R.L., Starita, R.J., and Poryzees, E.M., Argon laser trabeculoplasty in the treatment of secondary glaucoma. *Trans Am. Ophthalmol. Soc.*, 1983; 81: 325-32.

[7]   Logan, P., Burke, E., Joyce, P.D., and Eustace, P., Laser trabeculoplasty in the pseudo-exfoliation syndrome. *Trans. Ophthalmol. Soc. U K*, 1983; 103 (Pt 6): 586-7.

[8]   Horns, D.J., Bellows, A.R., Hutchinson, B.T., and Allen, R.C., Argon laser trabeculoplasty for open angle glaucoma. A retrospective study of 380 eyes. *Trans Ophthalmol. Soc. U K*, 1983; 103 (Pt 3): 288-96.

[9]   Strasser, G. and Witzmann, K., [Laser treatment for tightening the trabecular meshwork in open-angle glaucoma (trabeculoplasty)]. *Klin. Monbl. Augenheilkd.*, 1982; 181: 411-3.

[10]   The Glaucoma Laser Trial (GLT). 2. Results of argon laser trabeculoplasty versus topical medicines. The Glaucoma Laser Trial Research Group. *Ophthalmology*, 1990; 97: 1403-13.

[11] Parrish, J.A., Anderson, R.R., Harrist, T., Paul, B., and Murphy, G.F., Selective thermal effects with pulsed irradiation from lasers: from organ to organelle. *J. Invest. Dermatol.*, 1983; 80: 75s-80s.

[12] Murthy, S. and Latina, M.A., Pathophysiology of selective laser trabeculoplasty. *Int. Ophthalmol. Clin.*, 2009; 49: 89-98.

[13] Melamed, S., Pei, J., and Epstein, D.L., Delayed response to argon laser trabeculoplasty in monkeys. Morphological and morphometric analysis. *Arch. Ophthalmol.*, 1986; 104: 1078-83.

[14] Van Buskirk, E.M., Pathophysiology of laser trabeculoplasty. *Surv. Ophthalmol.*, 1989; 33: 264-72.

[15] van der Zypen, E. and Fankhauser, F., Ultrastructural changes of the trabecular meshwork of the monkey (Macaca speciosa) following irradiation with argon laser light. *Graefes Arch. Clin. Exp. Ophthalmol.*, 1984; 221: 249-61.

[16] Bylsma, S.S., Samples, J.R., Acott, T.S., and Van Buskirk, E.M., Trabecular cell division after argon laser trabeculoplasty. *Arch. Ophthalmol.*, 1988; 106: 544-7.

[17] Melamed, S., Pei, J., and Epstein, D.L., Short-term effect of argon laser trabeculoplasty in monkeys. *Arch. Ophthalmol.*, 1985; 103: 1546-52.

[18] Bradley, J.M., Anderssohn, A.M., Colvis, C.M., Parshley, D.E., Zhu, X.H., Ruddat, M.S., Samples, J.R., and Acott, T.S., Mediation of laser trabeculoplasty-induced matrix metalloproteinase expression by IL-1beta and TNFalpha. *Invest. Ophthalmol. Vis. Sci.*, 2000; 41: 422-30.

[19] Alvarado, J.A., Yeh, R.F., Franse-Carman, L., Marcellino, G., and Brownstein, M.J., Interactions between endothelia of the trabecular meshwork and of Schlemm's canal: a new insight into the regulation of aqueous outflow in the eye. *Trans Am. Ophthalmol. Soc*, 2005; 103: 148-62; discussion 162-3.

[20] Guzey, M., Vural, H., Satici, A., Karadede, S., and Dogan, Z., Increase of free oxygen radicals in aqueous humour induced by selective Nd:YAG laser trabeculoplasty in the rabbit. *Eur. J. Ophthalmol*, 2001; 11: 47-52.

[21] Kramer, T.R. and Noecker, R.J., Comparison of the morphologic changes after selective laser trabeculoplasty and argon laser trabeculoplasty in human eye bank eyes. *Ophthalmology*, 2001; 108: 773-9.

[22] Juzych, M.S., Chopra, V., Banitt, M.R., Hughes, B.A., Kim, C., Goulas, M.T., and Shin, D.H., Comparison of long-term outcomes of selective laser trabeculoplasty versus argon laser trabeculoplasty in open-angle glaucoma. *Ophthalmology*, 2004; 111: 1853-9.

[23] Latina, M.A. and de Leon, J.M., Selective laser trabeculoplasty. *Ophthalmol. Clin. North Am.*, 2005; 18: 409-19, vi.

[24] Melamed, S., Ben Simon, G.J., and Levkovitch-Verbin, H., Selective laser trabeculoplasty as primary treatment for open-angle glaucoma: a prospective, nonrandomized pilot study. *Arch. Ophthalmol.*, 2003; 121: 957-60.

[25] Liu, Y. and Birt, C.M., Argon Versus Selective Laser Trabeculoplasty in Younger Patients: 2-year Results. *J. Glaucoma*, 2011.

[26] Russo, V., Barone, A., Cosma, A., Stella, A., and Delle Noci, N., Selective laser trabeculoplasty versus argon laser trabeculoplasty in patients with uncontrolled open-angle glaucoma. *Eur. J. Ophthalmol.*, 2009; 19: 429-34.

[27]   Damji, K.F., Bovell, A.M., Hodge, W.G., Rock, W., Shah, K., Buhrmann, R., and Pan, Y.I., Selective laser trabeculoplasty versus argon laser trabeculoplasty: results from a 1-year randomised clinical trial. *Br. J. Ophthalmol.*, 2006; 90: 1490-4.

[28]   Martinez-de-la-Casa, J.M., Garcia-Feijoo, J., Castillo, A., Matilla, M., Macias, J.M., Benitez-del-Castillo, J.M., and Garcia-Sanchez, J., Selective vs argon laser trabeculoplasty: hypotensive efficacy, anterior chamber inflammation, and postoperative pain. *Eye (Lond)*, 2004; 18: 498-502.

[29]   The Glaucoma Laser Trial. I. Acute effects of argon laser trabeculoplasty on intraocular pressure. Glaucoma Laser Trial Research Group. *Arch. Ophthalmol.*, 1989; 107: 1135-42.

[30]   Barkana, Y. and Belkin, M., Selective laser trabeculoplasty. *Surv. Ophthalmol.*, 2007; 52: 634-54.

[31]   Harasymowycz, P.J., Papamatheakis, D.G., Latina, M., De Leon, M., Lesk, M.R., and Damji, K.F., Selective laser trabeculoplasty (SLT) complicated by intraocular pressure elevation in eyes with heavily pigmented trabecular meshworks. *Am. J. Ophthalmol.*, 2005; 139: 1110-3.

[32]   Rhee, D.J., Krad, O., and Pasquale, L.R., Hyphema following selective laser trabeculoplasty. *Ophthalmic. Surg. Lasers Imaging*, 2009; 40: 493-4.

[33]   Kim, D.Y. and Singh, A., Severe iritis and choroidal effusion following selective laser trabeculoplasty. *Ophthalmic. Surg. Lasers Imaging*, 2008; 39: 409-11.

[34]   Regina, M., Bunya, V.Y., Orlin, S.E., and Ansari, H., Corneal Edema and Haze After Selective Laser Trabeculoplasty. *J. Glaucoma*, 2010.

[35]   Weinand, F.S. and Althen, F., Long-term clinical results of selective laser trabeculoplasty in the treatment of primary open angle glaucoma. *Eur. J. Ophthalmol.*, 2006; 16: 100-4.

[36]   Van Buskirk, E.M., The laser step in early glaucoma therapy. *Am. J. Ophthalmol.*, 1991; 112: 87-90.

[37]   Popiela, G., Muzyka, M., Szelepin, L., Cwirko, M., and Nizankowska, M.H., [Use of YAG-Selecta laser and argon laser in the treatment of open angle glaucoma]. *Klin. Oczna*, 2000; 102: 129-33.

[38]   Mao, A.J., Pan, X.J., McIlraith, I., Strasfeld, M., Colev, G., and Hutnik, C., Development of a prediction rule to estimate the probability of acceptable intraocular pressure reduction after selective laser trabeculoplasty in open-angle glaucoma and ocular hypertension. *J. Glaucoma*, 2008; 17: 449-54.

[39]   de Leon, J.S., Dagianis, J.J., and Latina, M., Efficacy of Multiple Selective Laser Trabeculoplasty Treatments in Open Angle Glaucoma. *Invest Ophthalmol. Vis. Sci.*, 2005; 46.

[40]   Hong, B.K., Winer, J.C., Martone, J.F., Wand, M., Altman, B., and Shields, B., Repeat selective laser trabeculoplasty. *J. Glaucoma*, 2009; 18: 180-3.

[41]   Lai, J. and TE, B., Repeatability of Selective Laser Trabeculoplasty (SLT). *Invest. Ophthalmol. Vis. Sci.*, 2005; 46: E-Abstract 119.

[42]   Basile, M., Ostrovsky, A., Danias, J., Rothman, R., Prywes, A., Marcus, C., and Serle, J.B., Effect of third and fourth SLT on IOP. *Invest. Ophthalmol. Vis. Sci.*, 2008; 49: E-Abstract 1241.

[43] Lee, R. and Hutnik, C.M., Projected cost comparison of selective laser trabeculoplasty versus glaucoma medication in the Ontario Health Insurance Plan. *Can. J. Ophthalmol.*, 2006; 41: 449-56.

[44] Gulati, V. and Latina, M., Outcomes of Repeat Selective Laser Trabeculoplasty in Open Angle Glaucoma Cases on Medications. *Invest. Ophthalmol. Vis. Sci.*, 2004; 45: E-Abstract 5582.

[45] Buys, Y.M., Economics of selective laser trabeculoplasty as primary therapy for glaucoma. *Can. J. Ophthalmol.*, 2006; 41: 419-20.

[46] Leske, M.C., Connell, A.M., Schachat, A.P., and Hyman, L., The Barbados Eye Study. Prevalence of open angle glaucoma. *Arch. Ophthalmol.*, 1994; 112: 821-9.

[47] http://www.facebook.com/notes/st-lucia-blind-welfare-association/st-lucia-glaucoma-laser-project/118404514899076.

In: Glaucoma: Etiology, Pathogenesis and Treatments   ISBN: 978-1-61470-975-6
Editors: Z. G. Fei and S. Zeng   © 2012 Nova Science Publishers, Inc.

Chapter VI

The Parasurgical Treatment of Glaucoma

Felicia Ferreri, Pasquale Aragona, Giuseppina Ferreri and Giuseppe Ferreri
Universita' di Messina, Italy

ABSTRACT

The treatment parasurgical of glaucoma classically occupies an intermediate place between the medical and surgical therapy and it is frequently used when the patient's particular conditions or specific forms of glaucoma, do not allow surgery.

This type of therapy can be applied to the open-angle glaucoma (GPAA), acute glaucoma, and those glaucomas refractory to medical therapy and/or surgery.

PARASURGICAL THERAPY OF OPEN-ANGLE GLAUCOMA (GPAA)

The techniques used are two:

1. Laser therapy on the trabecular meshwork
2. Laser filtering trabeculotomy

1. Laser Therapy on the Trabecular Meshwork

The laser therapy in the treatment of trabecular meshwork in GPAA has been studied since 1979 by several authors with results that, at the beginning, were not completely encouraging. In 1979 Wise and Witter have codified the use of the Argon laser trabeculoplasty (ALT) in the treatment of GPAA [1].

The positive experience accumulated in more than 30 years of ALT indicate that this technique is always recommended to control the intraocular pressure (IOP) in GPAA before surgery and especially in those patients who, for various reasons, cannot stand the maximum medical therapy or who do not can be treated surgically.

The ALT, according to the guidelines by the European Glaucoma Society, is recommended in primary open angle glaucoma uncontrolled with medical therapy, pseudo-exfoliative glaucoma, pigmentary,glaucoma and in patients with poor compliance or intolerance to drugs.

In 1990, the Glaucoma Laser Trial [2] accomplished a randomized multicenter survey to evaluate the efficacy and safety of ALT as a first approach in the treatment of GPAA.

After two years of follow up, eyes treated with ALT, as initial therapy and which was possibly associated with topical therapy, had a lower mean IOP than eyes treated initially with topical therapy alone and also needed lower medications doses to control intraocular pressure. The contraindications essentially include a closed anterior chamber angle, opacity of dioptric media, that prevents the viewing of the angle structures and peculiar forms for GPAA.

The technique of ALT involves the use a gonioscopy contact lens (Goldmann (figure 1) or Ritch (Figure 2), CGA-lasag CH (Figure 3) applied with the interposition of methylcellulose after instillation of a mild miotic and of a surface anesthetic. It uses an argon laser and the parameters suggested by Wise and Witter are as follows: power 700-1200 mW, duration 0.1 sec, spot size 50 μm.

The spots should be aimed to the anterior part of the trabecular meshwork at the boundary between the pigmented and non-pigmented areas. The spots number should be of 50 in a space of 180 ° of trabecular meshwork.

The ideal reaction is given by the whitening of the trabecular meshwork with minimal bubbles formation [1]. The patient should continue antiglaucomatous therapy and the use of topical steroids for 5 days. Intraocular pressure was checked after 1, 24 hours, 7 and 30 days after the treatment.

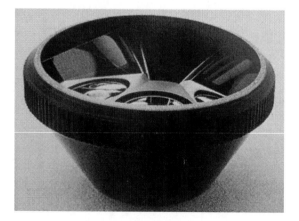

Figure 1.

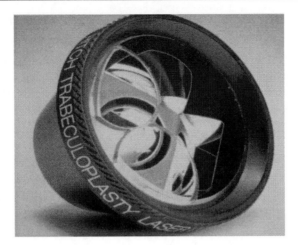

Figure 2.

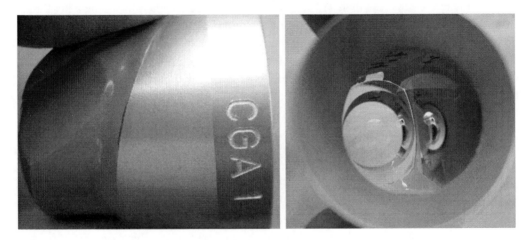

Figure 3.

Complications are rare, and include increased intraocular pressure [3], visual field reduction, pain, corneal burns, bleeding, peripheral anterior synechiae and iritis. The effectiveness of the technique is related to the initial pressure, lens condition, age, race, and type of glaucoma. The results are good in the short term and discrete in the long-term. The morphological alterations were studied on samples of human trabecular meshwork treated with ALT and collected in the course of trabeculectomy. [4] The alterations observed are similar to those seen in the eyes of monkey [5]. In the early phases there is a distribution of trabecular arches and an accumulation of cellular debris and fibrin; after 7 days there is a retraction of the uveal and corneo-scleral meshworks. After six months, areas of fibrosis and confluent endothelial cells lining the uveal trabecular meshwork and occluding its spaces, can be find. The reduction of intraocular pressure after ALT is caused by an increase aqueous outflow [6,7] not only due to scarring and subsequent reopening of the interlamellar spaces but especially to cellular changes such as increased mitosis and migration as well as a renewed extracellular matrix synthesis and turnover [2, 6,7,8,9]. A recently introduced technique is the Selective Laser Trabeculoplasty (SLT). This is selective photothermolysis [10], which uses a Q-switched, frequency doubled Nd: YAG laser, at 532 nm with a pulse duration of 3 nanoseconds. SLT selectively affects the pigment cells of the trabecular meshwork tissue without damaging the non-pigmented cells and the trabecular fibres. Comparative ultrastructural investigations have shown that with SLT the extent of the damage is minor compared with ALT [11]. The laser wavelength (532nm) is well absorbed by melanin, and therefore requires a minimum energy to obtain the cell stimulation. In fact, The SLT acts at the level of melanin granules, located in the cytoplasm of endothelial cells lining the trabecular spaces, resulting in a cavitation of cells. The result of this, is an intracellular cavitation damage, and the cell responds to injury by the upregulation of specific cytokines and the recruitment of macrophages that engulf the remaining cellular and extracellular melanin in the trabecolar network. Macrophages progressively widen and eventually reenter the blood circulation passing through the Schlemm's canal [12].

Besides the affinity between the wavelength of the laser and the pigment cells, the laser energy that is released is less than 1% of that required for ALT, and allows the use of a larger spot with a short application time. The result is a low fluence (energy/area) 6 vs 40,000 at a ratio of 1 / 6000. The heat dissipation and the photocoagulative damage both in the treatment areas and in the surrounding tissues is therefore limited. The effects of this treatment result is an increase of the aqueous outflow, after few hours, with the consequent decrease in intraocular pressure, and the appearance of new cells to maintain a long term reduction of the intraocular pressure. Numerous clinical studies have shown the efficacy and safety of SLT.

SLT complications are rare and include pain, inflammation, increased intraocular pressure, higher than ALT, in the early hours [13]. Six months after the treatment the results of the SLT technique are comparable to those obtained with ALT but with better safety: less anterior chamber inflammation, minor trabecular damage, equal duration of the hypotensive effect and equal efficacy in lowering IOP. The implementation of the SLT is relatively simple, is not even necessary to find the perfect angle structures. The procedure is executed, after instillation of topical anesthetic and application of gonioscopy lens, on 180-360 ° in one or two sessions (the second after one month). Fifty spots with a diameter of 400 μ, variable energy of 0.7-1.5 mJ, depending on the degree of pigmentation of the trabecular meshwork are the parameters applied. In conclusion SLT, is an interesting, alternative method to ALT, to be used as first treatment in GPAA [14,15].

2. Laser Filtering Trabeculotomy

The development of new types of lasers has made possible the realization of trabeculotomy through the sclera. The laser trabeculotomy have the advantage of being able to be performed in a short period of time and repeated several times. However, these techniques have poor circulation because the long-term results are very uncertain, either because they are subject to complications similar to those of filtration surgery (marked hypotonia, hyphema, low anterior chamber) or because corneal stroma and endothelium, iris and lens damages are often reported. The laser trabeculotomy can be performed both ab-external and internal. In the ab external procedure, the fistula is created beneath the conjunctiva by placing the laser fiber optic probe on the sclera just above the Schlemm's canal and the trabeculate. For this purpose can be used both the Holmium laser and the Excimer laser. The Holmium laser has been widely used in the Nineties. His laser beam, whose wavelength is near to the infrared, is entirely absorbed by water. a fiber optic probe is uses [16], which focuses the laser beam perpendicular to its axis, and the diameter of the spot at the tip of the probe is 200 μ. The probe is introduced 1-1,5 mm from the limbus and is advanced in the subconjunctival space to be positioned so that the emitted beam is applied on the sclera in the limbal area and directed in the anterior chamber. To pierce the sclera 6 to 50 pulses are needed, and the size of the fistula is usually 300 μ.

The excimer laser trabeculotomy (ELT) is a minimally invasive technique that reduces IOP. It can be performed as a stand-alone procedure or in combination with cataract surgery in just a few minutes. Laser spots are applied in the anterior chamber angle via an endoscopic camera lens or a gonio lens. In contrast to argon laser trabeculoplasty, shunts between the anterior chamber and Schlemm's canal are prepared by a laser photoablation. Thus, the outflow of aqueous humor will be improved. Best results can be expected in patients with moderately elevated intraocular pressure and cataract, undergoing the combined procedures.

Ab internal procedures are to create a fistula in departing from the anterior chamber. It is possible to use two techniques: 1) laser energy is directed through a goniolens on the sclera in the trabecular meshwork. 2) laser energy is applied directly to the sclera using a fiber optic probe that is introduced into the anterior chamber through a corneal or limbal incision and positioned against the sclera at the trabeculum.

PARASURGICAL THERAPY
OF THE ANGLE-CLOSURE GLAUCOMA

Laser iridotomy has now replaced surgical iridectomy in the treatment of acute glaucoma.

Where the attack of glaucoma is supported by a pupillary block, relative or absolute, creating an opening in the iris allows to match the blood pressure between the anterior and posterior chambers, so normalizing the pressure values provided that it is performed before the formation of irreversible peripheral synechiae. It is important to distinguish between the attack of glaucoma due to a pupillary block from that due to a plateau iris. The latter is characterized by an abnormal advanced insertion of the iris basis that may block the angle in course of mydriasis. In such cases there is no difference in the pressure between the anterior and posterior chambers, so that the laser iridotomy is ineffective, while it is more appropriate, together with the medical therapy, the laser gonioplasty, namely the expansion of the angle by the contraction of the peripheral iris stroma induced by the argon laser treatment. The indications to laser iridotomy are represented by the acute pupillary block glaucoma, the prophylaxis of acute glaucoma and in those cases where a deepening of the anterior chamber is needed. The contraindications are represented by all those conditions that do not allow precise visualization of the iris, such as corneal edema, and very low or absent anterior chamber. In performing a laser iridotomy it is appropriate that the patient is pretreated with the miotic agents to obtain a proper miosis. After instillation of local anesthetic, an Abraham's lens (figure 1),or Wise's lens (figure 2) or CGI LASAG CH lens (Figure 3), is applied to the cornea. This lens has the advantage of reducing by half the size of the spot, so the power and density of it increases by four times, thus facilitating the implementation of iridotomy. As to the location, the iridotomy is usually performed in the supero-nasal quadrant, close to the limbus and preferably at a crypt, in order to facilitate penetration. After the execution it is appropriate to prescribe the patient to use topical steroids for 3-4 days and check the intraocular pressure and the iridotomy after 24-48 hours. Laser iridotomy can be performed with argon laser, or more frequently with Yag laser (Figure 4) and the parameters are different depending on the type of laser used. With the argon can be used two ways:

1. Long-pulse technique (light Iris): spot diameter of 50 μ, power between 700 and 1500 mW, time of 0.2 sec and number of applications varying between 2 and 30.
2. Technique for short pulse (dark iris) is different than the previous technique for the time of impact of less than one-tenth, 0.02 sec, spot diameter of 50 μ, power between 1000 and 1500 mW and number of applications ranging from 50 to 100.

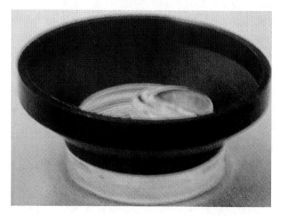

Figure 4.

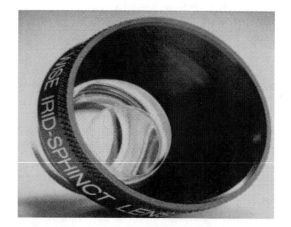

Figure 5.

The use of YAG laser in the execution of iridotomy has become popular also because the iridotomy performed with this technique have a much lower incidence of angle closure compared to those carried out with argon laser [9, 10]. It is used with an energy of 6.4 mJ and a burst of 3-4 impulses. Both lasers, YAG and argon, can be used together with a combined technique.

Argon is used in such cases to sculpt three-quarters of the iris surface, then the drilling of the iris is carried out with the YAG laser. This combined technique allows to create larger and more regular iridotomy (Figure 5). The backlight is not a reliable indicator of a completely perforated iris (Figure 6).

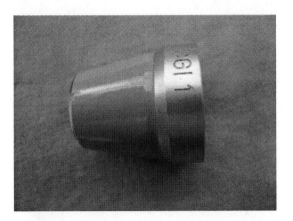

Figure 6.

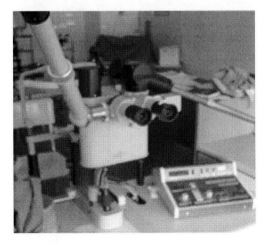

Figure 7.

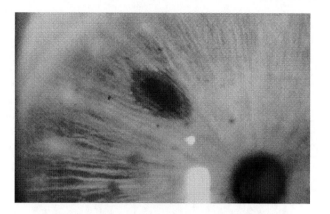

Figure 8.

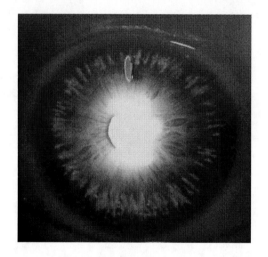

Figure 9.

Complications are represented by a progressive increase in the size of iridotomy with time, corneal burns, bleeding (especially with the YAG), increased intraocular pressure, and iritis posterior synechiae, localized opacity of the lens, diplopia, iridotomy closing late. [17,18,19,20].

PARASURGICAL THERAPY OF THE CILIARY BODY

The parasurgical techniques of the ciliary body are intended to reduce intraocular pressure by decreasing aqueous humor production. It is usually reserved for glaucoma refractory to other medical and surgical therapy. Therefore, it represents the ultimate therapy to be used in the treatment of incurable glaucoma, absolute glaucoma and in some painful secondary glaucoma (neovascular, post-traumatic). A number of techniques were proposed: the cyclo- diathermy the perforating cyclo- diathermy , the cyclo- photocoagulation, beta-irradiation[21], cyclo electrolysis[22] and the cyclo-cryotherapy [23]. All of these techniques, except cyclo cryotherapy and cyclo photocoagulation, permanently destroy the ciliary body and also cause serious complications (marked hypotonia, phthisis of the bulb) and, therefore, have been abandoned. The cyclo-cryotherapy is still used because it is less traumatic and has a much lower rate of serious complications. The technique is performed by transconjunctival via and involves the application of a cryoprobe tip, with the temperature of - 70 ° - 80 °, 3 mm far from the limbus. The application can be up to 180 ° or 360 °, and duration of application is 30 sec. The hypotensive effect is usually transient because the cyclo-cryotherapy does not cause necrosis of the ciliary body, but rather an anterior segment shock correlated to the reactive iridocyclitis caused by to the cold application [24]. Histological studies have shown at the level of the ciliary body intense vasodilation, edema and hemorrhage with necrosis [25]. Afterwards, a ciliary epithelium regeneration will determine a progressive increase of intraocular tension. However, with this technique is not possible to determine the treatment strenght so that, in case of over-dosage, it is frequent to observe severe bulbar hypotony and phthisis. Therefore, in order reduce side effects, techniques of treatment of the ciliary body with ultrasound and laser photocoagulation were proposed [25,26]. Cyclo-photocoagulation can be performed by transcleral, transpupillar and endoscopic application [27,28,29,30]. In transcleral cyclo-photocoagulation the energy of the YAG laser is brought to the ciliary processes through the sclera. It can be transmitted indirectly, no contact, or directly through optical fiber in contact with the eyeball.[31]In transcleral cyclo-photocoagulation is used both with the YAG laser, with wavelength of 1064 nm, which allows maximum penetration through the sclera (53%) with moderate absorption of melanin. both the diode laser , with a wavelength of 810 nm, which allows a scleral transmission slightly lower than the YAG, but with a better absorption of melanin. The parameters differ according to the method used. For the no contact method:

- YAG laser, output continuous or pulsed, energy 4-8 J/spot.
- Laser Diode; energy 1.5:-2 J 2 with a spot diameter of 100-400 μ

The technique provides 30-40 applications in a single session focusing 360 ° at 1-2 mm from the limbus. In the contact method, the laser can be coupled by an optical fiber that is applied perpendicular to the conjunctiva at 1.5 mm far from the limbus.

- The YAG laser energy for continuous emission spot 3.5-4 W, duration 0.5-0.7s, number of spots 16-40
- The laser Diode; energy 1.74-2,6W,duration 1.5-2.5 s, number of spots 16-20.

Positive results are achieved in approximately 60% of cases. The treatment is painful so it is necessary to perform peri or retro bulbar anesthesia.

The transpupillary cyclo-photocoagulation, described for the first time by Lee and Pomerantzeff in 1971, can be performed with argon laser, and is performed by focusing the laser energy, through the pupil in mydriasis, directly on the ciliary processes. This tecnique has a limited use due to the poor visualization of the ciliary processes (at least 1/3 should be clearly visualized) [32].

The endoscopic cyclo-photocoagulation, described by Shields el al in 1985, involves the use of Endolaser (argon laser) [33] and is considered a surgical technique because the instrument is introduced into the eye through the pars plana or the limbus. This tecnique provides a good view of the anatomical structure to be treated, using a lower energy consumption (power of 0.3 W for 1s) in about 60 spots. In 1995 Urami has associated this technique to phacoemulsification.

However, all these interventions on the ciliary body brings to inconsistent results, and all the cases results in iritis after treatment. The use of contact lasers may frequently induce edema and pain during the treatment; but the most serious complications are reported after the application of non contact lasers, in which the energy used is higher and the treated area is sometimes not clearly visible. Bulbar phtysis is reported in 10% of cases, persistent hypotonus in 26% and anterior chamber bleeding between 10-30%. The detachment of the choroid, sympathetic ophthalmia and hemovitreous are rare complications.

In conclusion, the techniques in the parasurgical treatment of glaucoma are many and varied and can be advantageously used when special conditions do not allow to perform surgery or in special forms of glaucoma refractory to other treatments.

In future, new laser sources will enable a further approach and better results, especially in the treatment of those glaucomas which are insensitive to any kind of medical or surgical therapy.

REFERENCES

[1]   Wise JB, Witter SLT: Argon laser therapy for open-angle glaucoma. A pilot study. *Arch. Ophthalmol.* 1979 Feb;97(2):319-22.
[2]   Glaucoma Laser Trial Research Group:The Glaucoma Laser Trial (GLT) and glaucoma laser trial follow-up study: 7. Results. *Am. J. Ophthalmol.* 1995 Dec;120(6):718-31.
[3]   Chen TC, Ang RT, Grosskreutz CL, Pasquale LR, Fan JT. :Brimonidine 0.2% versus apraclonidine 0.5% for prevention of intraocular pressure elevations after anterior segment laser surgery. *Ophthalmology.* 2001 Jun;108(6):1033-8.
[4]   Bylsma SS, Samples JR, Acott TS, Van Buskirk EM Trabecular cell division after argon laser trabeculoplasty. *Arch. Ophthalmol.* 1988 Apr;106(4):544-7.
[5]   Rodrigues MM, Spaeth GL, Donohoo P :Electron microscopy of argon laser therapy in phakic open-angle glaucoma. *Ophthalmology.* 1982 Mar;89(3):198-210.
[6]   Wilensky JT, Jampol LM:Laser therapy for open angle glaucoma. *Ophthalmology.* 1981 Mar;88(3):213-7.
[7]   Yablonski ME, Cook DJ, Gray J:A fluorophotometric study of the effect of argon laser trabeculoplasty on aqueous humor dynamics. *Am. J. Ophthalmol.* 1985 May 15;99(5):579-82.
[8]   Van Buskirk EM, Pond V, Rosenquist RC, Acott TS.:Argon laser trabeculoplasty. Studies of mechanism of action. *Ophthalmology.* 1984 Sep;91(9):1005-10.
[9]   Seiler T, Kriegerowski M, Bende T, Wollensak J.;Partial external trabeculectomy]. *Klin. Monbl. Augenheilkd.* 1989 Oct;195(4):216-20. German.
[10]   Latina MA, Park C.Selective targeting of trabecular meshwork cells: in vitro studies of pulsed and CW laser interactions. *Exp. Eye Res.* 1995 Apr;60(4):359-71.

[11] Cvenkel B, Hvala A, Drnovsek-Olup B, Gale N. Acute ultrastructural changes of the trabecular meshwork after selective laser trabeculoplasty and low power argon laser trabeculoplasty. *Lasers Surg. Med.* 2003;33(3):204-8.

[12] Guzey M, Vural H, Satici A, Karadede S, Dogan Z. Increase of free oxygen radicals in aqueous humour induced by selective Nd:YAG laser trabeculoplasty in the rabbit. *Eur. J. Ophthalmol.* 2001 Jan-Mar;11(1):47-52.

[13] Melamed S, Ben Simon GJ, Levkovitch-Verbin H.Selective laser trabeculoplasty as primary treatment for open-angle glaucoma: a prospective, nonrandomized pilot study. *Arch. Ophthalmol.* 2003 Jul;121(7):957-60.

[14] Weinand FS, Althen F, Long-term clinical results of selective laser trabeculoplasty in the treatment of primary open angle glaucoma. *Eur. J. Ophthalmol.* 2006 Jan-Feb;16(1):100-4.

[15] Latina MA, Tumbocon JA:Selective laser trabeculoplasty: a new treatment option for open angle glaucoma. *Curr. Opin. Ophthalmol.* 2002 Apr;13(2):94-6.

[16] Iwach AG, Hoskins HD Jr, Drake MV, Dickens CJ :Subconjunctival THC:YAG ("holmium") laser thermal sclerostomy ab externo. A one-year report. *Ophthalmology.* 1993 Mar;100(3):356-65; discussion 365-6.

[17] McAllister JA, Schwartz LW, Moster M, Spaeth GL.:Laser peripheral iridectomy comparing Q-switched neodymium YAG with argon. *Trans. Ophthalmol. Soc. U. K.* 1985;104 (Pt 1):67-9.

[18] Moster MR, Schwartz LW, Spaeth GL, Wilson RP, McAllister JA, Poryzees EM.:Laser iridectomy. A controlled study comparing argon and neodymium: YAG.*Ophthalmology.* 1986 Jan;93(1):20-4.

[19] Naveh-Floman N, Blumenthal M. A modified technique for serial use of argon and neodymium-YAG lasers in laser iridotomy. *Am. J. Ophthalmol.* 1985 Sep 15;100(3):485-6.

[20] Zadok D, Chayet A Lens opacity after neodymium: YAG laser iridectomy for phakic intraocular lens implantation. *J. Cataract. Refract. Surg.* 1999 Apr;25(4):592-3.

[21] Haik GM,Breffeilh LA,Barber A: beta irradiation as a possible therapeutic agent in glaucoma; an experimental study with the report of a clinical case. *Am. J. Ophthalmol.* 1948 Aug;31(8):945-52.

[22] Berens C, Sheppard Lb, Duel Ab Jr. Cycloelectrolysis for glaucoma. *Am. J. Ophthalmol.* 1951 Jan;34(1):53-70. No abstract available.

[23] Bietti G.:Surgical intervention on the ciliary body; new trends for the relief of glaucoma. *J. Am. Med. Assoc.* 1950 Mar 25;142(12):889-97.

[24] Boles Carenini B, Orzalesi N On the effects of cyclic cryotreatment on the function and ultrastructure of the ciliary body]. *Boll Ocul.* 1969 Mar;48(3):149-68.

[25] Scullica L, Pecori Giraldi J.Circulatory changes in the ciliary body after cryogenic therapy (preliminary research)]. *Boll Ocul.* 1969 May;48(5):302-11.

[26] Purnell EW, Sokollu A, Torchia R,Taner N.:Focal chorioretinitis produced by ultrasound.. *Invest. ophthalmol.* 1964 dec;3:657-64.

[27] Lee PF, Pomerantzeff O.: Transpupillary cyclophotocoagulation of rabbit eyes. An experimental approach to glaucoma surgery. *Am. J. Ophthalmol.* 1971 Apr;71(4): 911-20.

[28] Shields MB, Chandler DB, Hickingbotham D, Klintworth GK.Intraocular cyclophotocoagulation. Histopathologic evaluation in primates. *Arch. Ophthalmol.* 1985 Nov;103(11):1731-5.

[29] Brancato R, Leoni G, Trabucchi G, Trabucchi E.Transscleral contact cyclophotocoagulation with Nd:YAG laser CW: experimental study on rabbit eyes. *Int. J. Tissue React.* 1987;9(6):493-8.

[30] Wilensky JT, Welch D, Mirolovich M.Transscleral cyclocoagulation using a neodymium:YAG laser. *Ophthalmic. Surg.* 1985 Feb;16(2):95-8.

[31] Brancato R, Carassa RG, Bettin P, Fiori M, Trabucchi G.Contact transscleral cyclophotocoagulation with diode laser in refractory glaucoma. *Eur. J. Ophthalmol.* 1995 Jan-Mar;5(1):32-9.

[32] Brancato R, Giovanni L, Trabucchi G, Pietroni C.Contact transscleral cyclophotocoagulation with Nd:YAG laser in uncontrolled glaucoma. *Ophthalmic. Surg.* 1989 Aug;20(8):547-51.

[33] Crymes BM, Gross RL.Laser placement in noncontact Nd:YAG cyclophotocoagulation. *Am. J. Ophthalmol,* 108:456,1989.

In: Glaucoma: Etiology, Pathogenesis and Treatments   ISBN: 978-1-61470-975-6
Editors: Z. G. Fei and S. Zeng   © 2012 Nova Science Publishers, Inc.

Chapter VII

Effect of Synthetic Cannabinoid CB1 Agonist (WIN 55212-2) and Antagonist (AM 251) on Intraocular Pressure in Rats

Sergio Pinar-Sueiro[*1], *Rafael Rodríguez-Puertas*[2], *Iván Manuel*[3] *and Elena Vecino*[4]

[1]Department of Ophthalmology, Cruces Hospital.
Department of Cell Biology, University of the Basque Country, Vizcaya. Spain
[2]Department of Pharmacology. Department of Pharmacology,
University of the Basque Country, Vizcaya. Spain
[3]Department of Pharmacology, University of the Basque Country, Vizcaya. Spain
[4]Professor in Cell Biology. Department of Cell Biology,
University of the Basque Country, Vizcaya. Spain

ABSTRACT

Purpose: To study hypotensive effect of synthetic cannabinoid WIN 55212-2 when topically administered at 0.5% and 1% concentration. We also studied the normal distribution of CB1 receptors in ocular tissues from rats.

Matherials and controls: 24 female Sprague-Dawley rats, weighing between 250 and 300 g. Rats were divided in 6 groups according to the topical treatment for the left eye. Right eyes were considered as controls. Group 1: 0.5% WIN 55212-2, group 2: 1% WIN 55212-2, group 3: 0.5% AM 251, group 4: 1% AM 251, group 5: 0.5% AM 251 and 0.5% WIN 55212-2, and group 6: 1% AM 251 and 1% WIN 55212-2. Intraocular pressure was measured in awake animals with applanation tonometry. Afterwards, control right eyes were employed for immunohistochemistry for CB1 receptors.

* Corresponding author/adress for reprints: Sergio Pinar-Sueiro Department of Ophthalmology. Cruces Hospital. Plaza de Cruces s/n. CP: 48903 Vizcaya, Spain. Telephone number: +34 615 00 53 89 Fax number: +34 94 601 3266 E-mail address: luengonosvemos@yahoo.es

Results: WIN 55212-2 0.5% induced an average decrease of 4±2.5 mm Hg (or 23.86±15.04%), with respect to the corresponding right eye. WIN 55212-2 1% solution-treated eyes showed an average decrease of 6.8±2 mm Hg (or 37.10±9.98%), and there was less fluctuation in the IOP tendencies of the treated eyes, with respect to the corresponding right eye. Hypotensive effect is abolished by previously topically application of CB1 antagonist AM251. CB1 antagonist AM 251 showed no effect on IOP.

CB1 receptors were observed in the main therapeutic ocular targets for the treatment of glaucoma: trabecular meshwork, Schlemm`s canal, nonpigmented epithelium of the ciliar body, and retina.

Conclusions: WIN 55212-2 induce a dose-dependant intraocular hypotensive effect mainly through activation of CB1 receptors.

Keywords: WIN 55212-2, AM 251, cannabinoids, glaucoma, CB1 receptors, CB2 receptors, intraocular pressure, neuroprotection

SYNOPSIS

Synthetic CB1 agonist WIN 55212-2 induces a dose-dependent decrease on intraocular pressure (IOP), while cannabinoid antagonist AM 251 does not modify intraocular pressure by blocking the basal scarce effect of endocannabinoid interaction with CB1 receptors.

INTRODUCTION

Glaucoma is one of the leading causes of blindness worldwide. It consists on an optic neuropathy characterized by a progressive loss of retinal ganglion cells (RGCs). Clinically, this loss of RGCs represents typical patterns of perimetric defect or even reduced visual acuity. There are several known risk factors to develop glaucoma, and elevated intraocular pressure (IOP) is considered its major risk factor. Most treatments in glaucoma are directed to reduce this intraocular pressure in order to retard progression [1].

There's increasing evidence of the effect endocannabinoid system plays over the autorregulation of intraocular pressure. In the early 70's Hepler and Frank observed a reduction on IOP in subjects who smoked marijuana [2]. Merrit et al. probed the same effect with oral Δ^9-tetrahydrocannabinol (Δ^9-THC) [3], and Cooler and Gregg got a similar effect after intravenous administration of Δ^9-THC [4]. Some clinical studies have showed an important reduction of IOP in patients with glaucoma resistant to conventional therapies applying synthetic cannabinoids topically, and despite the difficulties to find the ideal dissolvent solution [5].

It was in the late 80's when the first cannabinoid receptor was identified in the rat brain [6], and, nowadays, we must talk at least of two major cannabinoid receptor subtypes, CB1 and CB2 [6, 7, 8]. The physiological mechanisms that are induced by the cannabinoid agonist, WIN 55212-2, to decrease the IOP are not well understood, although the described expression of mRNA for CB1 receptors in the ciliary processes and trabecular meshwork of the eye [9, 10, 11].

Therefore, the present work analyzes the time-course IOP in the rat eye when two different doses of the CB1 cannabinoid receptor agonist (WIN 55212-2) or the antagonist (AM 251), administered topically, diluted in a neutral and lipophylic solution. In adittion, the CB1 receptor localization is described by immunohistochemistry in the rat eye.

MATERIALS AND METHODS

Animals

We employed 24 female Sprague-Dawley rats, weighing between 250 and 300 g. The animals were cared with free access to food and water, at a stable temperature of 21°C and with a 12 h light-dark cycle. The Association for Research in Vision and Ophthalmology (ARVO) regulations for the care and treatment of animals subjected to ophthalmological experiments were adhered.

IOP Measurement in Awake Animals

Animals were kept awake and IOP measurements were followed for 3 days. The IOP of right and left eyes of awake animals was measuredusing planning tonometry (TonoPen XL, Mentor, Norwell, MA) after the application of tetracaine hydrochloride + oxibuprocaine (Coluircusí, Alcon Cusí, Barcelona, Spain). The tonometer was applied perpendicular to the more apical side of the cornea, until at least five or six independent measurements were obtained (each of these values was the average of four readings). The results of the IOP reading were accepted if the confidence interval was greater than or equal to 95% [12, 13].

Preparation of Eye Drop Solutions

WIN 55212-2 mesylate salt (Tocris Bioscience, Madrid, Spain) and AM 251 (Tocris Bioscience, Madrid, Spain) were dissolved in tocrisolve (Tocris, Madrid, Spain) solution. Final concentrations of 0.5 and 1% solutions of WIN 55212-2 and AM 251 were kept in borosilicate glass tubes previously treated with Sigmacote (SIGMA).

Treatment with WIN 55212-2 and AM 251

IOP was monitored before initiating experimental treatment. The 24 rats were divided into four groups. The right eye was always considered the control eye and was treated with the same frequency and volume with the solvent, Tocrisolve as placebo. The left eye was always the treated eye with 20 µl eyedrops at different concentrations.

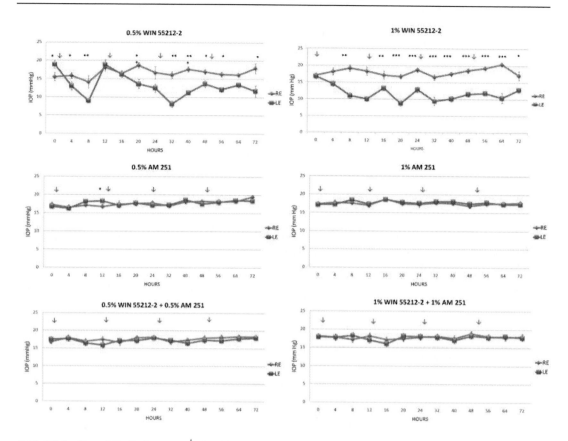

(RE: Right Eye; LE: Left Eye; ↓ Application of topical WIN 55212-2 and AM 251; *: p<0.05; **: p<0.005 significant reduction in mean IOP of treated eyes compared with contralateral vehicle-treated control eyes with 2-tailed paired t test).

Figure 1. Changes in intraocular pressure (IOP) following different topical treatments. Group 1 (n=4) animals were treated with multiple doses of topical 0.5% WIN 55212-2. Group 2 (n=4) animals were treated with multiple doses of topical 1% of topical WIN 55212-2. Animals in group 3 (n=4) and 4 (n=4) were treated with 0.5% and 1% topical AM 281, respectively. Animals in group 5 (n=4) were treated with 0.5% WIN 55212-2 and 0.5% AM251. Animals in group 6 (n=4) were treated with 1% WIN 55212-2 and 1% AM251. All treatments were performed on the left eye. Right eyes were considered as control eyes.

Group 1 (n=4) was topically treated with WIN 55212-2 at 0.5% solution every 12 hours for the first 24 hours (3 times), and one more eyedrop 24 hours later, in order to measure the biodisponibility of the drug. IOP measurements were done every 4 hours (Figure 1).

Group 2 (n=4) was treated with 1% solution of WIN 55212-2 and IOP was measured following the previous temporal protocol for group 1.

Group 3 (n=4) and group 4 (n=4) were topically treated with 20 µl of 0.5% or 1% AM251 solution, respectively, following the previous described temporal protocol.

Group 5 (n=4) was treated with 0.5% solution of AM 251 and 10 minutes later with 0.5% WIN 55212-2 and IOP was measured following the previous protocol.

Group 6 (n=4) was treated with 1% solution of AM 251 and 10 minutes later 1% WIN 55212-2 and IOP was measured following the previous temporal protocol.

Statistical Analysis

Statistical analysis was performed using SPSS software (SPSS Sciences, Chicago, IL). Intraocular pressure in different groups was expressed as mean +/- standard deviation. The mean values of IOP in different groups comparing treated and non-treated eyes were compared using one-way ANOVA test, followed by the Scheffé test. The minimum value of significant differences was defined as $p < 0.05$.

Immunohistochemistry

Control right eyes were employed for immunohistochemistry. Animals were anesthetized with chloral hydrate (400 mg/kg i.p.) and transcardially perfused by a cannula introduced into the ascending aorta. The cardiovascular system was washed with heparinized 0.9% NaCl at 37°C, and fixation was performed with 4% paraformaldehyde in phosphate buffer saline at 4°C (PBS 0.1M, pH 7.4). Eyes were removed and postfixed by immersion in the same cold fixative for 2-3 hours, followed by cryoprotection in a 3% sucrose solution for 8-12h. Tissues were frozen in isopentane at -80°C, and 12μm sections using a Microm cryostat at -25°C were done.

The primary antisera to the CB1 receptor (1:500) (anti-CB1: PA1-743, Affinity BioReagents, CO, USA), were diluted in PBS solution containing 0.5% of milk powder and bovine serum albumin (BSA) for blocking non-specific adsorption of the antibodies. Sections were washed by immersion for 15 minutes in phosphate buffer (0.1 M, pH 7.4) at room temperature and incubated overnight in the presence of the primary antibodies at 4°C. The tyramide signal amplification method was used to amplify the signal associated with the CB1 receptor antiserum. Briefly, sections were washed for 15 minutes in TNT buffer (0.1 M Tris, 0.15 M NaCl, 0.05% Tween 20, pH 7.5) and blocked in TNB solution (10 ml TNT buffer, 0.05 g blocking reagent, DuPont). Later on, sections were incubated with horseradish peroxidase (HRP) labelled donkey anti-rabbit secondary antibody (1:150) (Affinity BioReagents, CO, USA) for 30 min, followed by incubation with tyramide fluorescein (1:100, 10 min, room temperature). A Zeiss Axioskop 2 plus fluorescent light microscope was used for observation and digital photography of labelling in the slices.

RESULTS

WIN 55212-2 Solution

The mean basal IOP in the control right eyes (RE) of the first group was 16.7±1.24mm Hg. The mean IOP in WIN 55212-2 0.5% solution-treated left eyes was 12.8±2.87 mm Hg, with an average decrease of 4±2.5 mm Hg (or 23.86±15.04%), with respect to the corresponding right eye. A maximal reduction of 8±0,48 mm Hg (48.57±13.03%) was reached 8 hours after the second dose of 0.5% WIN 55212-2 solution.

The mean basal IOP in the right eyes of the second group was 18.1±1.16, and the mean IOP in WIN 55212-2 1% solution-treated eyes was 11.4±1.73 mm Hg, and there was less fluctuation in the IOP tendencies of the treated eyes, with an average decrease of 6.8 ± 2 mm Hg (or $37.10\pm9.98\%$), with respect to the corresponding right eye. A maximal reduction of 10 ± 3.46 mm Hg (or $49.40\pm18.04\%$) was reached 16 hours after third dose of 1% WIN 55212-2 solution.

AM 251 Solution

The mean basal IOP in the right eyes of the third group was 17.7 ± 0.80 mm Hg. The mean IOP in 0.5% AM 251 solution-treated left eyes was 17.7 ± 0.71 mm Hg. No statistical differences were observed between treated eyes and contralateral vehicle-treated eyes.

The mean basal IOP in the right eyes of the fourth group was 17.6 ± 0.45, and the mean IOP in 1% AM 251 solution-treated eyes was 17.8 ± 0.46 mm Hg, and there was less fluctuation in the IOP tendencies of the treated eyes. No statistical differences were observed between treated eyes and contralateral vehicle-treated eyes.

AM 251 Solution and WIN 55212-2

The mean basal IOP in the right eyes of the fifth group was 17.6 ± 0.62 mm Hg. The mean basal IOP in the eyes treated with 0.5% AM 251 solution and 0.5% WIN 55212-2 solution was 17.2 ± 0.64 mm Hg. No statistical differences were observed between treated eyes and contralateral vehicle-treated eyes.

The mean basal IOP in the right eyes of the fifth group was 17.9 ± 0.46 mm Hg. The mean basal IOP in the eyes treated with 0.5% AM 251 solution and 0.5% WIN 55212-2 solution was 17.7 ± 0.66 mm Hg. No statistical differences were observed between treated eyes and contralateral vehicle-treated eyes.

Biomicroscopic Analysis

Neither WIN 55212-2 nor AM 251 solutions' topical treatment showed no ocular side effects. No corneal/cristalline lens opacifications were seen, and no signs of inflammation in the anterior segment were observed at 0.5% as well as 1% concentrations used in the present study.

Immunohistochemistry

We found strong CB1 labeling in the ciliary nonpigment epithelium, corneal endothelium, trabecular meshwork and Schlemm`s canal, and outer segments of the photoreceptors. Moderate labeling was detected in the ciliary muscle, inner and outer nuclear and plexiform layers of the retina, as well as the retinal ganglion cell layer and nervous fiber layer (Figure 2, 3).

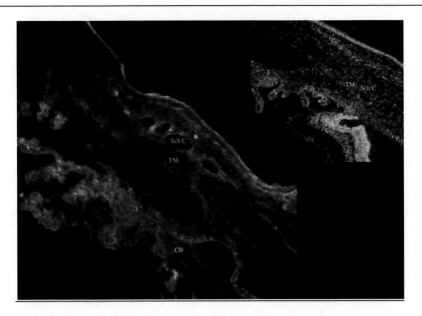

Figure 2. Immunohistochemistry of rat iridocorneal angle (x20). We find moderate to strong immunolabelling in the trabecular meshwork, schlemm canal, specially in the SCE cells and cells in the juxtacanalicular tissue (adjacent to SCE cells), and ciliar body. (Sch C: Schlemm canal; TM: Trabecular Meshwork; I: Iris; CB: Ciliar Body; SCE cells: Schlemm Canal's Endothelial cells).

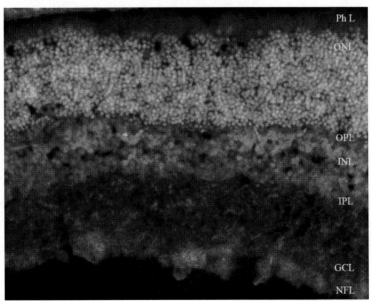

(Ph L: Photoreceptor Layer; ONL: Outer Nuclear Layer; OPL: Outer Plexiform Layer; INL: Inner Nuclear Layer; IPL: Inner Plexiform Layer; GCL: Ganglion Cell Layer; NFL: Nervous Fiber Layer).

Figure 3. Immunohistochemistry and DAPI labeling of rat retina (x20): Moderate CB1 receptor labeling is detected in the outer segments of the photoreceptors in the Ph L, ONL, location for the nuclei and cell bodies of the rod and cone cells, INL, constituted by cell bodies and nuclei of bipolar and horizontal cells, synapses between bipolar cell processes and dendritic processes of ganglion cells in the IPL, cell bodies of ganglion cells of the GCL and in the axonal fibers from the ganglion cells (NFL).

Systemic Side Effects

Apparently, WIN 55212-2 and AM 251 topical application didn't induce any systemic adverse effects. After topical application of both drugs animals resumed their standard locomotor activity almost inmediatelly. No significant differences in weight increase/loss were observed between rats in different groups.

DISCUSSION

WIN 55212-2 is a synthetic aminoalkylindole that mainly binds to CB1 cannabinoid receptor, but also it has been described a partial bind to CB2 receptors [14]. Previous studies showed a dose-dependent reduction over IOP in normal monkeys after topical application of eyedrops of WIN 55212-2 [14]. However, according to that study 0,5% concentration reached barely any further effect over IOP than 0,2% concentration, considering this concentration as the maximum dose to apply topically. In our study, 0.5% concentration of WIN 55212-2 solution gets a significant decrease of IOP in the eyes in which treatment is applied compared with the contralateral, however, its effect is not as constant as 1% WIN 55212-2 solution. Thus at 1% concentration, IOP remains low with less fluctuation, reaching this constant 24-hours effect even only with a sole application daily.

The mechanism by which cannabinoids reduce IOP is not yet known. It has been suggested to act directly as vasodilators of the efferent blood vessels of the anterior uvea, improving outflow [5]. Some studies have demonstrated that by acting through CB1 and CB2 receptors, cannabinoid agonists modulate the trabecular meshwork cell actin's cytoskeleton and migration, enlarging the spaces between cells, which could mediate in the decrease of intraocular pressure [15, 16]. It has also been proved that topical application of WIN 55212-2 decreases IOP both in normal and glaucomatous monkey eyes mainly by decreasing aqueous flow [14]. Our present study showed intraocular hipotensive effect of WIN 55212-2 was mediated through CB1 receptors, as this effect of decreasing intraocular pressure was neutralized by a CB1 the receptor antagonist AM 251.

Despite the effect on IOP played by cannabinoid receptor agonists, cannabinoid antagonist barely showed effect on IOP when topically administered.

In previous studies, Laine et al. demonstrated that topical administration of AM 251 blocked the reduction of IOP induced by CB1 agonists [17]. AM251 has very low affinity for the CB2 cannabinoid receptor (350-fold selectivity for CB1 compared to CB2 receptors) and is considered an inverse agonist of CB1 receptors. A plausible explanation for the lack of effect on IOP of AM 251 should be the poor role of endocannabinoids over aqueous humor basal production over ciliary processes, as well as a reduced effect on modulating the trabecullar meshwork cell's migration, compared to the IOP lowering effect when activating same type of receptors with more potent synthetic cannabinoid receptor agonists (WIN 55212-2).

This study gives more strength to the possibilities of CB1 agonists as topical treatment for glaucoma; however, further studies should determine the applicability of CB1 agonist eyedrops in the daily clinical practice.

ACKNOWLEDGMENTS

We are grateful for support from The Glaucoma Foundation (TGF; USA), Spanish Ministry of Science and Technology (SAF2007-62060), Grupos Consolidados del Gobierno Vasco, RETICS, Fundación Jesús Gangoiti Barrera, Red Patología Ocular RD07/0062, ONCE, BIOEF08/ER/006.

REFERENCES

[1]   The AGIS Investigators. The Advanced Glaucoma Intervention Study (AGIS): 7. The relationship between control of intraocular pressure and visual field deterioration. The AGIS Investigators. *Am. J. Ophthalmol.* 2000; 130:429-440.

[2]   Hepler RS, Frank IM. Marihuana smoking and intraocular pressure. *JAMA* 1971; 271:1392.

[3]   Merrit JC, McKinnon S, Armstrong JR, et al. Oral Δ^9-tetrahydrocannabinol in heterogeneous glaucomas. *Ann. Ophthalmol.* 1980; 12:947-950.

[4]   Cooler P, Gregg JM. The effect of delta-9-tetrahydrocannabinol on intraocular pressure in humans. *South Med. J.* 1977; 70:951-954.

[5]   Porcella A, Maxia C, Gessa GL, et al. The synthetic cannabinoid WIN 55212-2 decreases the intraocular pressure in human glaucoma resistant to conventional therapies. *Eur. J. Neurosci.* 2001; 13(2):409-412.

[6]   Devane WA, Dysarz FA III, Johnson MR, et al. Determination and characterization of a cannabinoid receptor in rat brain. *Mol. Pharmacol.* 1988; 34:605-613.

[7]   Munro S, Thomas KL, Abu-Shaar M. Molecular characterization of a peripheral receptor for cannabinoids. *Nature* 1993; 365:61-65.

[8]   Devane WA, Hanuš L, Breuer A, et al. Isolation and structure of a brain constituent that binds to the cannabinoid receptor. *Science* 1992; 258:1946-1949.

[9]   Stamer WD, Golightly SF, Hosohata Y, et al. Cannabinoid CB1 receptor expression, activation, and detection of endogenous ligand in trabecular meshwork and ciliary process tissues. *Eur. J. Pharmacol.* 2001; 431:277-286.

[10] Porcella A, Casellas P, Gessa GL, Pani L. Cannabinoid receptor CB1 mRNA is highly expressed in the rat ciliary body: implications for the antiglaucoma properties of marihuana. *Mol. Brain Res.* 1998; 58:240-245.

[11] Straiker AJ, Maguire G, Mackie K, Lindsey J. Localization of cannabinoid CB1 receptors in the human anterior eye and retina. *Invest. Ophthalmol. Vis. Sci.* 1999; 40:2442-2448.

[12] Urcola JH, Hernández M, Vecino E. Three experimental glaucoma models in rats: comparison of the effects of intraocular pressure elevation on retinal ganglion cell size and death. *Exp. Eye Res.* 2006; 83(2):429-437.

[13] Hernández M, Urcola JH, Vecino E. Retinal ganglion cell neuroprotection in a rat model of glaucoma following brimonidine, latanoprost or combined treatments. *Exp. Eye Res.* 2008; 86(5):798-806.

[14] Chien FY, Wang R-F, Mittag TW, Podos SM. Effect of WIN 55212-2, a cannabinoid receptor agonist on aqueous humor dynamics in monkeys. *Arch. Ophthalmol.* 2003; 121(1):87-90.

[15] Kumar A, Song Z-H. CB1 cannabinoid receptor-mediated changes of trabecular meshwork celular properties. *Mol. Vis.* 2006; 12:290-297.

[16] He F, Song Z-H. Molecular and cellular changes induced by the activation of CB2 cannabinoid receptors in trabecular meshwork cells. *Mol. Vis.* 2007; 13: 1348-1356.

[17] Laine K, Järvinen D, Mechoulam R, et al. Comparison of the enzymatic stability and intraocular pressure effects of 2-arachidonylglycerol and noladin ether, a novel putative endocannabinoid. *Invest. Ophthalmol. Vis. Sci.* 2002; 43:3216-3222.

Index

F

G

H

T

U

V

W

Z